ESSENTIAL SKILLS FOR A MEDICAL TEACHER

An Introduction to Teaching and Learning in Medicine

Second Edition

Ronald M. Harden OBE MD FRCP (Glas) FRCPC FRCS (Ed)

Professor Emeritus Medical Education, University of Dundee, UK,
General Secretary, Association for Medical Education in Europe (AMEE)
Editor, Medical Teacher

Jennifer M. Laidlaw DipEdTech MMEd

Formerly Assistant Director, Education Development Unit, Scottish Council for Postgraduate Medical and Dental Education at the University of Dundee, Dundee, UK

Foreword by

David M. Irby PhD

Professor of Medicine, University of California, San Francisco, USA

ELSEVIER Edinburgh London New York Oxford Philadelphia St Louis Sydney Toronto

ELSEVIER

ISBN: 978-0-7020-6958-1
Printed in China
Last digit is the print number: 9 8 7 6 5 4 3 2 1

Content Strategist: Laurence Hunter
Content Development Specialist: Carole McMurray
Project Manager: Anne Collett
Design: Christian Bilbow
Illustration Manager: Amy Faith Heyden
Illustrator: MPS North America, LLC

ELSEVIER your source for books, journals and multimedia in the health sciences

www.elsevierhealth.com

  Working together to grow libraries in developing countries

www.elsevier.com • www.bookaid.org

The publisher's policy is to use paper manufactured from sustainable forests

Contents

Foreword   ix

Preface   xi

About the Authors   xiii

Acknowledgements   xv

SECTION 1 The 'Good Teacher'   1

1 The teacher is important   3

2 The different faces of a good teacher   9

3 Understanding basic educational principles   15

4 Being an enthusiastic and passionate teacher   27

5 Knowing what works best   33

6 Collaborating and working as a team   41

7 Checking your performance as a teacher and keeping up to date   49

SECTION 2 What the Student Should Learn   55

8 The move to an outcome/competency-based approach   57

9 Specifying the learning outcomes and competencies   67

10 Describing and communicating the learning outcomes and competencies   73

11 Implementing an outcome-based approach in practice   81

SECTION 3 Curriculum Development   87

12 The 'authentic' curriculum   89

13 Ten questions to ask when planning a curriculum   95

14 Sequencing curriculum content and the spiral curriculum   103

15 Student engagement and a student-centred approach   109

16 Building learning around clinical problems and presentations   117

17 Using an integrated approach   125

18 Interprofessional education (IPE)   131

19 The apprenticeship, community-based education, longitudinal clinical clerkships and work-based learning   135

20 Responding to information overload and building options into a core curriculum with threshold concepts   145

21 Recognising the importance of the education environment   153

22 Mapping the curriculum   159

SECTION 4 Styles of Teaching   165

23 The lecture and teaching with large groups   167

24 Learning in small groups   175

25 Independent learning   183

26 Teaching and learning in the clinical context   189

27 Simulation of the clinical experience   195

28 E-learning   203

29 Peer and collaborative learning   211

SECTION 5 Assessment   217

30 Six questions to ask about assessment   219

31 Written and computer-based assessment   231

32 Clinical and performance-based assessment   237

33 Portfolio assessment   247

34 Assessment for admission to medicine and postgraduate training   253

35 Evaluating the curriculum   259

1 Entrustable Professional Activities (EPAs) for undergraduate medical education as specified by the Association of American Medical Colleges (AAMC) 268

2 The learning outcomes for a competent practitioner based on the three-circle model 269

3 Four dimensions of student progression 271

4 A page from a study guide, 'Learning paediatrics: a training guide for senior house officers' 272

5 Summary of various points in the continuum between a problem-based approach and an information-oriented approach 273

6 The clinical presentations that provide a framework for the curriculum in task-based learning 275

7 First two sections of the learning outcome/tasks mastery grid for vocational training in dentistry 277

8 Dundee Ready Education Environment Measure (DREEM) 278

9 Examples of OSCE stations 279

Index 281

CONTENTS

Foreword

The other night I was watching my favorite team play an amazing game of basketball. In the last seconds of the game, the most valuable player lobbed the ball from mid court while running flat out and being aggressively pursued by opponents to make the basket and win the game. I cheered for this stunning achievement, which appeared so easy to perform. More recently I watched an especially gifted and enthusiastic physician teach a team of learners in the hospital. I was equally amazed by her skills at engaging her team in thinking through a complex patient case, framing and guiding the inquiry process, and eloquently adding insights about treatment options along the way. It was a joy to behold and appeared to be performed with seamless effort and grace.

Expertise, in the form of basketball and clinical teaching, appears to be performed in a fluid and effortless manner. Yet, in both instances, these different forms of expertise required thousands of hours of deliberate practice to achieve this level of excellence and grace. To achieve such performance requires high levels of practice with a focus on improvement. By deliberate practice I mean conscious and effortful working on the component parts of expertise to improve them and then moving forward to tackle additional components – always striving for greater levels of competence.

I have observed and worked with many faculty members who wished to improve their teaching and engaged in deliberate practice. When their commitment to change was matched with repetitive practice, coaching and resources, they made exceptional progress. I have seen the worst rated teacher in a clinical department turn into a highly rated teacher – receiving the resident golden apple award for the most improved teacher. I have also worked with faculty members who had no desire to improve their teaching. My recommendations for improvement went unheeded and their dreadful teaching continued unabated. So, there must be both a commitment to change and reflective practice or no change will occur and it will be a waste of everyone's time.

For those who are interested in improving their own teaching and increasing the range of instructional options available to them, this book can serve as a practical guide. It is a treasure trove of tips on instruction, curriculum and assessment, and should be of special interest to those who are struggling with their own teaching or with a particularly challenging learner or who merely want to expand their repertoire of teaching skills.

Teaching is often learned through the apprenticeship of experience – through watching others and reflecting on one's own teaching. This can result in either excellent or poor teaching practices – depending on the role models available and the reflective capacity of the teacher. Fortunately, there is more to go on than these idiosyncratic forms of experience. There is a growing evidence-base about human learning, teaching, curriculum and assessment. This book offers evidence-based guidance for teaching that facilitates learning. Strategies highlighted in the book offer a broad range of options for teaching and learning.

Since teaching is based on scripts that guide content selection and teaching activity, the longer teachers provide instruction the more routinized their teaching becomes. This automation results in cognitive efficiency but it also makes change more difficult. This might suggest a strategy for reading this book. One way to approach the book is to read it from cover to cover, like a good novel. While this will offer an overview, relatively little will be retained in memory, assimilated into existing teaching scripts and utilized to improve teaching. Another way to read the book is to see it as a consultant – someone to ask for help in solving a particular instructional problem. Read to learn how to reframe a problem and create a new approach to addressing it. In other words, when trying to change a long established habit or script, focus on one or two new behaviors, experiment with them and repetitively practice them until automation is achieved. Then move on to try something new.

Yet, teaching is more than a set of skills; it is also a relational process in which the teacher embodies the best qualities of being a teacher and clinician. Sharing passion and enthusiasm for teaching and patient care can have a profound affect on learning. Such excitement is infectious. In addition, if learners sense that teachers have their best interests at heart, they not only appreciate the teaching but are more tolerant of less than stellar teaching practices. For example, teachers who ask difficult questions of learners at the bedside can be perceived as either being supportive and fostering learning or as being hostile and abusive. Caring for learners matters.

Clinical teachers can also have a profound influence on the learning climate of the work setting. In clinical environments where participation is learning, a welcoming stance toward learners can make all the difference. A positive learning climate is built upon teacher enthusiasm and humility, welcoming and respectful relationships, and a balance of challenge and support. Learning within such groups is motivating, engaging and enjoyable – no matter the workload. Inviting learners into the work and supporting their participation is critical to effective learning.

In addition to gleaning practical tips for teaching improvement from this book, think about how to create your own learning community. Who else shares your passion for teaching improvement? Create a learning community with another person, small group or department. Review chapters together and discuss the application of the concepts and strategies to your own teaching. In addition, collaborative learning processes can be achieved at national or international meetings. Faculty development programs and academies of medical educators can also offer learning communities and can create new networks of colleagues and educators.

This book offers insights and inspiration as well as essential skills for the medical teacher. Enjoy the read and share it with others.

David M. Irby, PhD

Professor of Medicine and Member of the Office of Medical Education, University of California, San Francisco School of Medicine, San Francisco, CA, USA.

Preface

Since the publication of the first edition of *Essential Skills for a Medical Teacher*, which was well received and highly commended by the British Medical Association, medical education has continued to evolve in response to improvements in healthcare delivery, advances in medical practice, changes in patient expectations and developments in education thinking and technology. This second edition reflects on these developments and the move from theory to practice and to a more authentic curriculum based on the real world rather than on an 'ivory tower.'

Although the need for expertise in teaching has been recognised for some time, there has been increasing appreciation since the first edition was published that all charged with the responsibility of serving as teachers or trainers in medicine have a personal responsibility to acquire the necessary education understanding and skills to allow them to meet the demands placed on them.

It is an exciting time for teachers and trainers, with greater collaboration possible between medical scientists and clinicians, between teachers locally, nationally and internationally, and between those engaged with the different undergraduate, postgraduate and continuing phases of education. Be prepared also for students to become partners in the education process and not simply as the consumers.

In this new edition we have three aims. The first is to provide the reader with practical hints and guidelines that will help him or her to create powerful learning opportunities for their students. We have not been overprescriptive, recognising that readers will need to adapt the recommendations to suit their own situations.

Our second aim is to introduce some key basic principles that underpin the practical advice given and help to inform teaching practice. Concepts such as the FAIR principles for effective learning were a feature of the first edition and proved helpful to the readers. These have been retained and strengthened.

Effective teaching demands much more than the acquisition of technical skills. An understanding of these principles is essential if the teacher is to be able to respond to the changes that have taken place in the learning context and to the continuing demands for change.

Our third aim is to assist readers to reflect on and analyse with colleagues the different ways that their work as a teacher or trainer can be approached and how their students' or trainees' learning can be made more effective. What makes teaching exciting is that each situation is different. Through responding to this challenge, teachers will achieve more satisfaction and enjoyment in their work.

Expect to be introduced to new ideas, such as the 'flipped classroom', Entrustable Professional Activities, the longitudinal clerkships, threshold concepts and the curriculum cube. Learn about the advantages of having an authentic curriculum, the value of teamwork and interprofessional education, and the continued development of outcome- or competency-based education. There is also a greater emphasis on performance assessment, curriculum mapping and a more seamless transition across the different phases of the education programme with students introduced to patients from the first year of the curriculum.

There are five sections in the book and at the beginning of each one you will find a summary of the key messages and new trends and developments. The information and suggestions offered are based on our extensive experience in teaching and curriculum planning and in the organisation of faculty development courses in medical education at basic and advanced levels.

At the end of each chapter you are invited to reflect on your own teaching practice and react accordingly. There are also additional references that enable you to delve deeper into the topics being covered.

We have considered the great constraints placed on teachers' and trainers' time and for this reason we have kept the book succinct. It was Albert Einstein who said that 'any intelligent fool can make things bigger and more complex'. We hope we have avoided doing so.

Whatever your role is in the training of tomorrow's doctors, whether it be in undergraduate, postgraduate or continuing education, or whether you are a novice or an experienced teacher, we hope you will find this book both enjoyable and useful.

Ronald M. Harden
Jennifer M. Laidlaw

About the Authors

Ronald M. Harden

Professor Ronald Harden graduated from the medical school in Glasgow, UK. He completed training and practised as an endocrinologist before moving full time to medical education. Professor Harden was Professor of Medical Education, Teaching Dean, Director of the Centre for Medical Education and Postgraduate Dean at the University of Dundee. He is currently editor of *Medical Teacher* and General Secretary and Treasurer of the Association for Medical Education in Europe (AMEE).

Professor Harden is committed to developing new approaches to medical education, curriculum planning, and teaching and learning. Ideas that he has pioneered include the Objective Structured Clinical Examination (OSCE), which has been universally adopted as a standard approach to assessment of clinical competence. He has published more than 400 papers in leading journals and is co-editor or co-author of the books *A Practical Guide for Medical Teachers*, the *Definitive Guide to the OSCE* and the *Routledge International Handbook of Medical Education*. He has also lectured and run courses on medical education across the globe.

His contributions to excellence in medical education have attracted numerous awards, including honorary fellowships of the Royal College of Physicians and Surgeons of Canada and the Royal College of Surgeons in Edinburgh, the Hubbard Award by the National Board of Medical Examiners in the USA, the MILES award by the National University of Singapore, the Karolinska Institutet Prize for Research in Medical Education, the ASME Richard Farrow Gold Medal, the AMEE Lifetime Achievement Award, an honorary MD degree, Tampere, Finland and the Cura Personalis Honour, the University of Georgetown's highest award, USA. In addition he was awarded the OBE by the Queen for his services to medical education.

Jennifer M. Laidlaw

Jennifer Laidlaw joined the University of Dundee's Centre for Medical Education in 1975 having previously been a media resource officer for the Royal Bank of Scotland and an innovator of their first distance learning programmes for bank staff.

At the University of Dundee she initially taught on a Diploma in Medical Education course attended by WHO fellows from the Eastern Mediterranean Region (EMRO).

For over 20 years she planned, organised and led courses on medical education both in Dundee and overseas.

She has acted as a medical education consultant for the World Health Organisation, the British Council, medical schools and colleges. She has run workshops in Malaysia, the United Arab Emirates, Australia, Egypt, Kuwait, Thailand, Bangladesh, Hungary and Romania.

She provided the educational design for the Centre's distance learning programmes, which were distributed to over 50 000 healthcare professionals, including general practitioners, surgeons, pharmacists, dentists, nurses and physiotherapists. Her postgraduate experience was with junior doctors, designing and teaching on induction courses.

She initiated the Twelve Tips series, which continues to be produced by the journal *Medical Teacher*, and provided the educational design for the series Developing the Teaching Instinct produced by the Education Development Unit of the Scottish Council for Postgraduate Medical and Dental Education.

In her teaching, whether it be face-to-face or at a distance, she has applied the FAIR principles that are highlighted in this book. The approach has certainly worked for her.

Acknowledgements

The understanding and experiences in medical education which we share in this book have been gained and made immeasurably richer through our association with former colleagues Len Biran, Jack Genn, staff of the Centre for Medical Education in Dundee, the late Miriam Friedman Ben-David and the late Willie Dunn. They have brought to medical education unique perspectives from which we have benefited. We are grateful to all who have shared their experiences and views on medical education with us at conferences, through papers we have read, and in schools we have visited. We have learned a lot working with the excellent facilitators on our Essential Skills in Medical Education (ESME) courses and from the participants who have shared their thoughts with us. Medical education is an applied discipline and only by seeing and experiencing at first hand what works and what does not work have we been able to distil what we believe to be helpful advice.

We are grateful to David Irby, who has written the foreword to this book, and the team at Elsevier, in particular Laurence Hunter and Carole McMurray, for their practical help and advice. Jim Glen drew the cartoons, which we hope both entertain the reader and help convey the messages.

SECTION 1

The 'Good Teacher'

'Good teachers are enthusiastic and enjoy teaching. Their enthusiasm for teaching and their subject is infectious.'

Jane Dacre, 2003

- The teacher is key to the success of an education programme
- The role of the teacher in the education process is changing
- The 'good' teacher has the necessary technical skills and an appropriate approach to their teaching that includes an understanding of basic educational principles to facilitate learning, an appropriate attitude and passion for their teaching, appropriate decision-making strategies and excellent collaboration skills
- Teachers take personal responsibility for evaluating their performance and for their continued professional development as a teacher
- The necessary attributes required of the teacher can be learned. 'Poor' teachers can become 'good' teachers and 'good' teachers can become 'excellent' teachers

The teacher is important 1

Teachers have an important influence on the students' experience of the education programme, their achievement of the learning outcomes and the sort of doctor they become.

The curriculum, the student and the teacher

The educational process has three elements: the curriculum, the student and the teacher (Figure 1.1). Much attention has been paid to the curriculum, including the different approaches to teaching, learning and assessment, and to students, including their selection for admission to medical studies and how they can learn more effectively. Less attention has been paid to the teacher. The teacher or trainer, however, is a key element in the creation of the conditions in which learning occurs. (We have used interchangeably throughout the book 'teacher' or 'trainer' and 'student' or 'learner'.) Lawrence Stenhouse, an education guru, suggested that there could be no such thing as curriculum development without teacher development. Good teachers have a range of technical skills, an understanding of basic educational principles, an enthusiasm and passion for teaching and a commitment to evaluating and improving their own teaching. The possession of these attributes by a teacher is important.

Thomas Good (2010), reviewing research on teaching, illustrated the importance of the teacher, using the analogy of how a chicken dinner with salad, wine and an apple can be a completely different experience as we move from restaurant to restaurant or eat at different homes. While the meal can always be improved by better wine or new ingredients, more important is how the basic ingredients are prepared and presented. As Good outlined, the literature on effective teaching is

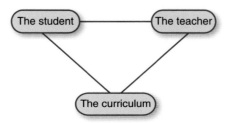

Figure 1.1 The three elements in the education programme

not based on evidence showing that the most effective teachers bring in new components or better ingredients. Rather the literature indicates that some teachers work with basic ingredients better than others. More important than the method of teaching is how it is implemented in practice by the teacher and the student–teacher interaction.

The teacher matters

The teacher is critical to the success or failure of the education programme – to the planning and implementation of the curriculum, to the student's learning and to the assessment of the student's progress. This applies when new approaches such as team-based learning or the flipped classroom are introduced and to the use of more traditional methods such as the lecture. There are, as we discuss in Chapter 23, no bad lectures only bad lecturers.

Teachers in fact are the medical school or postgraduate body's greatest asset. Dan Tosteson, former Dean at Harvard, suggested that the most important thing we as teachers have to offer our students is ourselves. There is overwhelming evidence that the quality of the teacher makes a huge difference to the effectiveness and the efficiency of the student's learning. More than half a century ago, Sir Derrick Dunlop wrote in 1963 in a publication *The Future of Medical Education in Scotland*, 'It is important to remember that the actual details of the curriculum matter little in comparison to the selection of students and teachers. If these are good any system will work pretty well; if they are indifferent the most perfect curriculum will fail to produce results.' This is equally true today. Teaching, like a clinical skill, is important – if you don't get it right it can have other serious implications.

Accrediting bodies, such as the General Medical Council in the UK, have recognised that all doctors to a greater or lesser extent have teaching responsibilities, and have highlighted teaching competence as an important learning outcome in undergraduate and postgraduate programmes. A teacher, to fulfil their educational role, needs to possess or acquire the necessary knowledge, skills and attitudes. If you are a teacher, a trainer, a clinical supervisor, someone with responsibility for a section of a course or a dean, you can make a difference to the quality of your students' or trainees' learning experience. *A European Union High Level Group: Train the Professors to Teach* recommended, 'All staff teaching in higher education institutions in 2020 should have received certified pedagogical training. Continuous professional education as teachers should become a requirement for teachers in the higher education sector.'

The necessary attributes can be learned

Over the past two decades significant changes have taken place in how the doctor of tomorrow is trained and, as indicated in the Preface, medical education continues to evolve. Some of these changes are outlined in Table 1.1. The status quo in education is not an option. The *Lancet* report 'Health professionals for a new century: transforming education to strengthen health systems in an independent

Table 1.1 Changes in medical education

Past	Present
Emphasis on the process and the methods of teaching and learning	Emphasis on the product and the learning outcomes
Learning dominated by mastery of basic and clinical science theory	Authentic learning with theory related to real-life situations and problems
Clinical experiences introduced later in the course	Clinical experiences introduced early in the course
Learning through lectures and hospital-based clinical teaching	A mixed economy including e-learning and simulation and learning in ambulatory and community-based settings
Teachers take responsibility for the education	Students actively engage in their own learning
A uniform or standard education programme	Teaching personalised to the needs of individual students
Curriculum content compartmentalised and discipline-based	Curriculum content integrated
Education focused on the medical profession	Interprofessional education and learning to work in teams
A competitive environment with students learning as individuals	Students collaborating and learning together
Assessment prioritises mastery of fact	Assessment rewards application of knowledge, skills and attitudes
Emphasis on being correct, with mistakes and errors ignored	Learning from mistakes and errors in practice
Education decisions made on the teacher's prejudice and personal experience	Education decisions informed by the best evidence available

THE TEACHER IS IMPORTANT

world' (Frenk et al. 2010) argued that 'Professional education has not kept pace with these challenges, largely because of fragmented, outdated, and static curricula that produce ill-equipped graduates.' The Flexner follow-up report by the Carnegie Foundation *Educating Physicians: A Call for Reform of Medical Schools and Residency* (Cooke et al. 2010) and the Canadian report *The Future of Medical Education in Canada (FMEC): A Collective Vision for MD Education* (AFMC 2010) also advocated the need for changes in medical education programmes. These changes impose new demands on the teacher. They require of the teacher, as described in this book, a more informed understanding and a new set of skills.

It is now recognised that expertise in medicine or in a content area is not necessarily associated with the skills required to teach the subject to students or trainees. While a good teacher may have naturally the necessary skills and passion to teach others, some of the required skills have to be learned. Everyone can learn to be a teacher. In teaching, much may be seen as common sense or obvious but experience shows that when it comes to putting it into practice, teachers often flounder and are found wanting. Teachers can learn from experience but this in itself is not enough. This point is illustrated when we look at golfers who go round a golf course practising their mistakes but if the mistakes are never rectified the golfer is unlikely to improve.

There is no magic bullet to becoming a competent teacher but this book points you in the right direction. The book addresses four key questions:

- what should be learned or taught (the learning outcomes)
- how the training or learning programme is organised (the curriculum)
- how students or trainees learn most effectively (the teaching and learning methods)
- how the learning and the student's progress is assessed (assessment).

Teaching is a personal matter. The commitment of teachers and trainers is important if they are to respond adequately to the challenges facing medical education. The work should be enjoyed and not endured. Whether you are working with students in the undergraduate curriculum or with trainees in postgraduate or specialist training we hope the chapters that follow will help you find that teaching well is more fun and satisfying than teaching poorly. The book has been written in the belief that teaching is both a craft and a science and that, with a better understanding of their work, 'poor' teachers can become 'good' teachers and 'good' teachers can become 'excellent' teachers.

Motivation for teaching

Many medical schools and institutions now recognise good teaching with financial incentives or promotion. Good teaching can bring its own rewards and perhaps the greatest reward is knowing that through teaching you as a teacher are helping to shape the next generation of doctors. Christa McAuliffe was to be the first teacher in space but died tragically when her spaceship disintegrated 70 seconds after take-off. Earlier, when asked what she did, she had replied, 'I touch the future, I teach.'

A teacher's personal motivation to teach was found by Dybowski and Harendza (2014) to comprise a range of factors from intrinsic, such as the joy of teaching itself, to more extrinsic motives, such as the perception of teaching as an occupational duty. Faculty-specific structures, such as curriculum organisation, hierarchies, differential aspects of leadership and human resource development, as well as evaluation systems and incentives, also played a prominent role.

Over to you

Reflect and react

1. Is your contribution as a teacher important to your students?
2. Look at the education changes summarised in Table 1.1. How do these impact on your role as a teacher?
3. What additional knowledge or skills might help you in your work as a teacher?

Explore further

Journal articles

Dybowski, C., Harendza, H., 2014. 'Teaching is like nightshifts ...': a focus group study on the teaching motivations of clinicians. Teach. Learn. Med. 26, 393–400.

Feinberg, N.R., Koltz, E.F., 2015. Getting started as a medical teacher in times of change. Med. Sci. Educ. 25, 69–74.

A personal view of teaching in medicine.

Frenk, J., Chen, L., Bhutta, Z.A., et al., 2010. Health professionals for a new century: transforming education to strengthen health systems in an interdependent world. Lancet 376, 1923–1958.

An authoritative report on the changes needed in medical education.

Tosteson, D.C., 1979. Learning medicine. N. Engl. J. Med. 301, 690–694.

Reports

AFMC, 2010. The Future of a Medical Education in Canada (FMEC): a collective vision for MD education. The Association of Faculties of Medicine of Canada, Ottawa.

A vision for the developments of medical education in Canada.

Dunlop, D., 1963. Medical education in Scotland. In: Goldberg, A. Future of Medical Education in Scotland. Scottish Medical Journal, Glasgow.

The importance of the teacher.

Books

Cooke, M., Irby, D.M., O'Brien, B.C., 2010. Educating Physicians: A Call for Reform of Medical School and Residency. Jossey–Bass, San Francisco.

A review of medical education in the USA.

Good, T.L., 2010. Forty years of research on teaching 1968–2008: What do we know now that we didn't know then? In: Marzano, R.J. (Ed.), On Excellence in Teaching. Solution Tree Press, Bloomington, IN, pp. 31–64.

*Good teachers and trainers are much more than transmitters of
information and skills. They facilitate students' learning and
they do this in a number of ways. Technical competence and how
teachers approach their work are both important.*

What is required of a good teacher

Teachers today have a challenging and multi-faceted role. Teaching is about much
more than the transmission of information to the learner. Teaching encompasses
the tasks of planning, preparing and delivering a learning programme and assessing
whether students have achieved the expected learning outcomes. Students learn all
of the time. It is a natural activity. The job of a teacher is to facilitate this by working
with the students to:

- clarify the expected learning outcomes
- deliver a programme with appropriate learning opportunities
- support and facilitate the student's learning
- assess the learner's progress in achieving the set goals.

An analogy, in some respects, is the travel agent who, with special knowledge in an
area, provides clients with information about their destination according to their
specific requirements, assists them to explore the range of options that match their
needs, arranges the necessary transport and accommodation, and advises on a programme of activities at their destination.

What is required of the teacher is demanding. Teaching, Brookfield (1990) suggested,
is the 'educational equivalent of white water rafting'.

The good teacher embodies a range of abilities

Teaching is a complex activity that requires the teacher to have a range of abilities. This includes not only mastery of the content area but also the technical
competencies necessary to serve as an information provider, a role model, a facilitator of learning, a curriculum planner, an assessor, a manager and a scholar. As

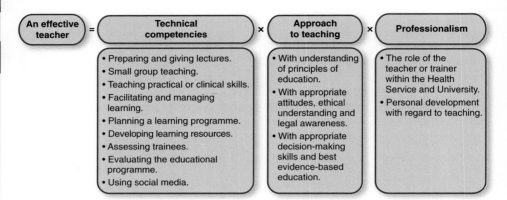

Figure 2.1 The competencies and attributes expected of an effective teacher

a professional, the teacher requires a basic understanding of the underpinning educational principles and an appropriate attitude and passion for teaching. If you have the necessary skills, teaching is not a chore; it can be an enjoyable experience and can be rewarding and fun. The good teacher will have a passion for teaching that will help to motivate and inspire students and trainees. The teacher should be an enquirer into his or her own competence and should keep up to date with developments in the field.

The attributes of a good teacher are summarised in Figure 2.1. Here lies a problem. Staff development programmes and texts on the subject frequently address only the technical competencies, or alternatively focus on the educational theory, which may be seen by the practising teacher as of little relevance. The concept of professionalism and attitudes to teaching are largely ignored. It is now recognised that the effective teacher requires, as shown in the figure, a combination of technical competence, an appropriate approach to their teaching, and professionalism in their work as a teacher. These are described in more detail in the chapters that follow.

The multiplication symbol has been used in the equation in Figure 2.1 rather than the addition symbol. The implication is that a demonstration of technical competence, no matter how good, on its own is not sufficient. A zero score for the approach to teaching or for professionalism will result in a total score for the teacher of zero.

Teaching is both an art and a science. Some teachers are instinctively good teachers but others are not. The reassuring fact, however, is that the art and science of teaching can be learned. The experienced teacher can develop further their teaching instinct and the new teacher can be helped to acquire this instinct and the necessary competencies, attitudes and professionalism.

What is required of a good teacher will vary to some extent depending on the subject being taught, and in which part of the world the teaching is taking place. There are, however, certain principles, approaches and views of teaching that are common to the different contexts. We highlight these in this book. It can be argued that the similarities are greater than any differences.

The technical competencies of a good teacher

Nine core areas of technical task-orientated competencies for a teacher are described in Figure 2.1.

A teacher should be competent in:

- preparing and giving lectures or presentations that engage the audience and make use of appropriate technology
- choosing appropriate small group methods and facilitating a small group teaching session
- teaching practical or clinical skills in a variety of settings including the work place
- facilitating and managing the student's learning in a range of settings, giving the learner support to obtain the maximum benefit from the learning opportunities available, helping the student to assess his or her own competence and providing feedback to the learner as necessary
- planning an education programme for the students or trainees that combines appropriate learning opportunities to help them to achieve the expected learning outcomes
- identifying, developing and adapting learning resources for use by students in the form of handouts, study guides or multimedia presentations
- assessing the achievement of learning outcomes by the students or trainees using appropriate technologies including written, performance-based and portfolio assessments
- evaluating the education programme, including the use of feedback from the learner and peer assessment
- using social media.

A question to be asked is in how many of these skills does a teacher need to be highly proficient? Depending on the local circumstances, the required level of mastery of the skills may vary. It can be argued that a level of understanding and basic level of proficiency in all of the skills is necessary.

When teachers are asked in how many of these competencies they would expect a good teacher to excel, the answers vary from all of the competencies to a smaller number.

How a good teacher approaches their work

An effective teacher, in addition to having the necessary technical competencies, approaches teaching with:

- *An understanding of basic educational principles*

    As discussed in Chapter 3, an understanding of basic educational principles helps teachers to adapt the teaching approach to their own situation, to deal with problems and difficulties encountered, and to respond to the need for change as it arises.

- *Appropriate ethics and attitudes*

    The ethical standards expected of medical teachers in their work as a teacher or researcher in medical education has been a focus of attention. As discussed in Chapter 4, the teacher's attitude is about much more than ethical behaviour. A key factor in student learning is a teacher's attitude, passion and enthusiasm for the subject and for their teaching.

- *Strategies for decision making*

    Paralleling the move to evidence-based medicine, the need for the teacher to make education decisions informed by the best evidence available is very much on today's agenda. At the same time, the good teacher has to be able to behave intuitively and to respond appropriately to unexpected situations as they arise in the classroom or workplace learning situation. This is discussed in Chapter 5.

The good teacher as a professional

Teachers as professionals should be enquirers into their own competence, should reflect on their own teaching practice, and should audit the quality of their teaching. Teachers have the personal responsibility to keep themselves up to date with current approaches to teaching, and to communicate their own experiences and lessons learned to others. This is discussed in Chapter 7. An excellent teacher will successfully innovate in the teaching domain and contribute to the development of new courses and curriculum reform.

Writing in *Scholarship Reconsidered*, Boyer (1990) described teaching as one of the scholarships expected of faculty or staff in a university.

Over to you

Reflect and react

1. How effective a teacher are you in terms of your technical competencies as summarised in Figure 2.1?
2. A doctor has an understanding of the medical sciences and how the body works. As a teacher have you an understanding of basic educational principles to ensure learning can be made more effective?
3. Do you convey to your students a passion for your subject and demonstrate an enthusiasm for their learning?
4. Have you a commitment to assess your own competence as a teacher and to keeping yourself up to date?

Explore further

Journal articles

Harden, R.M., Crosby, J.R., 2000. AMEE Educational Guide No. 20. The good teacher is more than a lecturer – the twelve roles of the teacher. Med. Teach. 22, 334–347.

A description of the twelve roles of the medical teacher grouped into six areas.

Hatem, C.J., Searle, N.S., Gunderman, R., et al., 2011. The educational attributes and responsibilities of effective medical educators. Acad. Med. 86, 474–480.

Hesketh, E.A., Bagnall, G., Buckley, E.G., et al., 2001. A framework for developing excellence as a clinical educator. Med. Educ. 35, 555–564.

A description of the twelve areas of competence expected of a clinical teacher.

Srinivasan, M., Li, S.T., Meyers, F.J., et al., 2011. 'Teaching as a competency': competencies for medical educators. Acad. Med. 86, 1211–1220.

Reports

Boyer, E.L., 1990. Scholarship Reconsidered: Priorities of the Professoriate. John Wiley and Sons, New York.

The classic text that recognised teaching as a scholarly activity.

Books

Brookfield, S., 1990. The Skilful Teacher, p2. Jossey–Bass, San Francisco.

A description of what is expected of the teacher

Sotto, E., 1994. When Teaching Becomes Learning. Cassell, London.

An account of good teaching practice and associated theoretical concepts based on scholarly sources.

A teacher is a professional not a technician. An understanding of some basic principles about learning can inform the teacher or trainer in their day-to-day teaching.

Be FAIR to your students

A good teacher, as we have discussed in the previous chapter, does not operate using a cookbook approach, blindly following a set of rules or procedures. Good teaching, just like any other field of professional endeavour, is best delivered when there is an understanding of the underlying process. Educational researchers have devoted a lifetime to studying education and have described a variety of theories and factors that influence learning (Taylor and Hamdy 2013). The work in educational psychology described in educational textbooks is often more associated with the experimental laboratory than the reality of practice in the classroom. There are, however, some basic general principles about learning that can inform what we do as medical teachers.

A comprehensive study of educational theory is out of place in this book and in any case is unlikely to be of interest or relevance to the reader. We have distilled four key principles about effective learning to which teachers can relate in their day-to-day practice. By applying these principles you will improve the effectiveness and efficiency of learning and this can lead to a better learning experience for the student or trainee. Most learners in the healthcare professions are capable learners and should have little difficulty in achieving the expected learning outcomes providing they are given some help from their teacher or supervisor.

We have used the acronym FAIR (see Figure 3.1). Be FAIR to your students by providing:

Feedback. Give feedback to students as they progress to mastery of the expected learning outcomes.
Activity. Engage the student in active rather than passive learning.
Individualisation. Relate the learning to the needs of the individual student.
Relevance. Make the learning relevant to the students in terms of their career objectives.

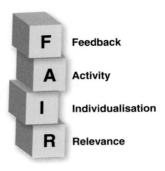

Figure 3.1 The FAIR principles for effective learning

The theme that runs throughout this chapter and other chapters in the book is that if we have a better understanding of how students learn and apply the FAIR principles in our teaching programme, gains in the student's performance will result. Students are naturally motivated to learn. 'The problem', suggests Sotto (1994), 'appears to be to find a way of teaching which does not inhibit motivation and to find a way of teaching which is in line with the motivation already present in the learners.' One answer is to apply the FAIR principles. In the right conditions, students can take more responsibility for their own learning. This is discussed further in Chapter 15. Application of the FAIR principles helps to create these conditions.

Since we first described the FAIR model for effective learning the model has been applied with benefit to the learner in a wide range of contexts in undergraduate, postgraduate and continuing education around the world. These include student learning in the early years of the course, work-based learning in clinical rotations and in the community, the Objective Structured Clinical Examination (OSCE) and other approaches to assessment, and new developments in teaching such as the flipped classroom and peer teaching.

Feedback

Feedback can be thought of as information communicated to the learner that is intended to modify his or her thinking or behaviour in order to improve learning. Satisfaction studies carried out both with undergraduate students and postgraduate trainees have revealed that one of the commonest complaints students have is that they do not receive meaningful feedback. Too often feedback is omitted or, if provided, is not seen to be helpful.

Feedback provided by the teacher to the student serves a number of functions:

- Feedback provides a basis for correcting mistakes. It enables learners to recognise their deficiencies and helps to guide them in their further study.
- Feedback clarifies learning goals. It highlights what is expected of the learner.
- Feedback reinforces good performance. It has a motivating effect on the learner and may reduce anxiety.

Feedback is part of a two-way communication between a teacher or trainer and the learner, and will provide for learners an insight into their performance that they might not otherwise have. Knowledge by the learner of the extent to which they have achieved the expected learning outcomes can lead to more effective and efficient learning. It has been demonstrated that academic achievement in classes where effective feedback is provided for students is considerably higher than in classes where this is not so. Hattie and Timperley (2007) argued that the most powerful single thing that teachers can do to enhance achievement of their students is to provide them with feedback.

How to give constructive feedback has been identified by teachers as one of the core competencies thought to be important in their work as a teacher. Much is known about how effective feedback can be provided. It is a skill that can be learned. Here we provide evidence-based practical guidelines that if put into practice will help you to improve your students' learning.

- *Make feedback part of the institutional culture.* Try to create a climate for the educational programme where feedback is expected and valued and where it occurs regularly. The quality of the feedback process should be monitored by the institution. The feedback should be seen as part of an interactive process between the teacher and the student, where there is mutual trust and respect.
- *Feedback should be timely and time should be set aside to provide students with feedback.* Feedback is more effective when learners receive it immediately than when it is delayed and provided in a later class or session. We have found for example that providing students with feedback in a session immediately following an OSCE is a useful and powerful learning experience (Harden et al. 2016). Feedback should be scheduled at a time in the course when the student has the opportunity to respond by engaging in activities designed to remedy any deficiencies identified.
- *Prepare adequately in advance.* Ensure that you have all the available evidence with regard to the students' performance before you attempt to provide them with feedback. The teacher should be in a position to provide feedback from first-hand experience with the student. This is preferable to basing feedback on second-hand reports.
- *The learner should understand what it is they are expected to achieve from the feedback session.* Some learners may find it difficult to accept and act on feedback provided. One strategy that has been shown to help is to ask the learner, before the actual content of the feedback is considered, to reflect orally or in writing on their attitude to being given the feedback.
- *Give an explanation that is specific and related to the expected learning outcomes.* Provide students with an explanation of what they did or did not do to meet the expectations. Simply giving a grade or mark in an examination or indicating that learners are right or wrong is less likely to improve their performance. The aim is to help the learner reflect on their performance and to understand the gaps in their learning. Provide learners with feedback about their performance against clearly defined learning outcomes. Informing

learners how they compare to their peers or informing them in general terms that they lack competence in an area is of little value.

- *Feedback should be non-evaluative.* Feedback should be descriptive and phrased in as neutral or non-judgemental language as possible. It is not helpful, for example, to inform learners that their performance was 'poor' or 'totally inadequate'.
- *Feedback should be part of a two-way collaboration between student and teacher.* Feedback should not be seen as a one-way process with the teacher providing the learner with comments and advice.
- *Feedback should help learners to plan their further study.* Conclude with an action plan and assist learners to plan their programme of further learning based on their understanding of where they are at present. This may involve giving them specific reading material or organising further practical or clinical experiences appropriate to their needs.
- *Incorporate peer feedback.* Students learn more effectively when feedback is provided from peers as well as from teachers. In a continuing professional development programme, general practitioners were provided with feedback about their management of a series of patient scenarios (Harden et al. 1979). Feedback from colleagues was found to be valued more highly than feedback from experts. Multi-source feedback (MSF) and the role of peers, colleagues and patients in assessment is discussed further in Chapter 32.
- *Encourage learners to provide feedback to themselves.* Feedback is usually thought of as something that is provided exclusively by teachers. Students should be encouraged to assess and monitor their own performance. Ask the learners whether they think they have done well and where they think there are problems. Learners can be provided with tools to assist them to assess themselves. Following an OSCE, for example, students can be given a copy of their marked OSCE checklist, a video of their performance and a video demonstrating the expected performance at the OSCE station (Harden et al. 2016).

Provision of feedback is important and is particularly difficult in the 'problem' learner when the learner is achieving significantly below their potential. Coupled with early recognition and appropriate intervention, effective feedback is essential if a trainee in difficulty is to be managed effectively and successfully.

Activity

A second strategy that has been shown to enhance achievement is to actively involve the students and trainees in the learning. The principle of active learning is implicit in many of the changes that have taken place in the medical curriculum. These include student-centred approaches, problem-based learning, team-based learning, the use of small group work and, as described in Chapter 23, the 'flipped classroom'. The traditional lecture has been criticised as too passive, with information being passed from the lecturer's notes to the student's notes without going through the brain of either.

Evidence demonstrates that where a learner is actively involved in the learning process, the achievements will be significantly enhanced. There is no doubt that students learn best when they are actively engaged in mastering a clinical skill or acquiring new knowledge. Learners should be challenged to think and review what they are studying and how new information and skills can be incorporated into their existing knowledge base and skills repertoire. This active learning results in a deeper and more meaningful processing of the learning material, with information being stored in the long-term memory.

In active learning, students take ownership of the learning and are encouraged to reflect and to think critically about what they are learning. Reflection is a key part of active learning (Sandars 2009). Time should be set aside to enable students to reflect on their experiences and gain a new understanding. What we need to guard against is 'inert knowledge' – information transmitted to the student that is not used and is usually forgotten.

Active learning can be encouraged by asking the student to:

- Gain new knowledge or understanding of a topic by activating their prior knowledge and building on what they already know
- Apply their knowledge to a new problem or patient presented to them
- Test their understanding through a self-assessment exercise. This may be a set of multiple choice questions or clinical scenarios
- Carry out a procedure, e.g. using a simulator
- Reflect on their experience in order to gain a new understanding and appreciation as documented, for example, in a portfolio
- Share their knowledge with other students. In peer learning, both the peer tutor and the tutee benefit.

Some learning methods, such as simulation or portfolio learning, by their very nature actively engage the student while others such as the lecture or the standard printed text are frequently associated with passive learning. Almost all learning situations, however, can be transformed from a passive to an active one. This is the challenge for the teacher. Here are some examples:

- Where *lectures* are scheduled, engage the audience by asking them to reflect on and respond to what is being discussed. An electronic audience response system with a 'clicker', an online survey tool, or coloured cards can be used as described in Chapter 23. The students may be asked to tackle or answer a problem in discussion with other students next to them.
- *Small group teaching*, as described in Chapter 24, by its nature is more interactive but guard against it regressing into a mini tutorial. Learners should actively engage with other group members and with the teacher who acts as the facilitator of the discussion rather than the presenter of information – 'the guide on the side rather than the sage on the stage'.
- In the *clinical context* ensure that learners are not simply passive observers of the patients and the events in the ward or clinic. Learners can be given

specific roles and be encouraged to be actively involved in a patient care activity.

- *Independent learning* resources recommended for use by students, whether in print or online, should also be interactive. Available texts or resources can be enriched by the teacher through the addition of meaningful activities that actively engage the student.
- *Simulations and virtual patients provide rich opportunities for active learning.* Support material in the form of print, audio recordings, videos or online programmes can be provided to assist learners to use these resources. Activities may be programmed into the simulator.
- Ensure that *portfolios* involve an active reflection process and are not simply a log or rote documentation of activities carried out by the learner. Work on a portfolio should not be seen as a chore but rather an opportunity for learners to reflect on the task and document what they have learned in the process.

Whatever the context – whether in the lecture theatre, small group situation, practical laboratory, clinical setting or independent learning – it is essential that activities scheduled are designed to be meaningful and not divert the student from the learning goals. Clicking to turn a page in an e-learning programme is an activity but it does not contribute to the student's learning. It is important that the teacher and students grasp the purpose or function of an activity and how it contributes to a mastery of the learning outcomes.

The development of student activities by the teacher can be time-consuming but also rewarding. The associated cost and resource implications can be justified more easily where the object of the learning is a complex task, such as management of a patient with diabetes, or a difficult concept, such as gaining an understanding of acid–base balance.

Individualisation

In the present consumer culture, the needs of the individual are being increasingly recognised whether it is in relation to planning a holiday or purchasing a computer to meet the user's personal requirements or expectations. In London, we see advertisement boards that adjust their display to the characteristics of the person approaching, e.g. an older man in a suit or a young more casually dressed woman. Large stores are experimenting with the use of intelligent price labelling that adjusts the sale price depending on whether the person approaching has a store loyalty card or has previously purchased goods. A new car stereo system promises to create personalised sound in the car that allow four occupants to listen to different music or to take telephone calls without other passengers being able to hear. In medicine too we see a personalised approach, with the management of patients matched to their personal needs.

The situation in education, however, is very different. Students, like patients, all have different needs and learn in different ways, but in most medical schools

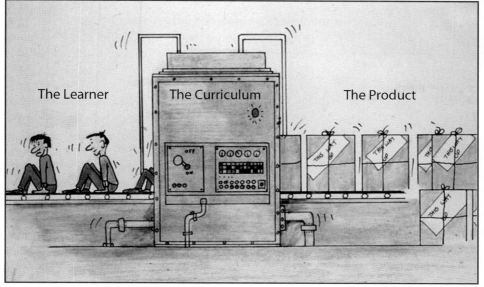

Figure 3.2 A factory approach with a standard product

teachers cope with large classes of students and have designed the learning experiences and programmes accordingly. As illustrated in Figure 3.2, students, like the raw material entering a factory, pass through a standard process emerging as a product with a uniform specification. There has been little opportunity to cater for the needs of the individual student, although some attempts may be made to do so.

Students have different requirements in terms of:

- personal capabilities
- motivation and what drives their learning
- learning goals and career aspirations
- levels of mastery of the course learning outcomes on entry to the course
- learning styles
- the place of learning – on campus or at a distance
- the time available for learning.

Students are now less willing to accept teaching and learning opportunities that do not match their needs and help them to achieve their personal learning goals. With the availability of new learning technologies, we need to work towards an 'adaptive learning' programme where the experience offered to students adapts to their personal needs as they work through the programme. Of the four principles described in this chapter, individualisation is probably the most difficult to apply. It is the one where we are likely to see the most change in the next decade with a move to a more adaptive curriculum where learning experiences are tailored to the needs of the individual student. This is described further in Chapter 15.

Students and trainees acquire knowledge and competencies at different rates. For this reason we also see a move from a curriculum where **time is fixed** for the students to study a subject or gain experience and what is **variable is the standard students achieve**, to a curriculum where the **standard is fixed** and what is **variable is time**.

We will see the development of adaptive learning both at the level of the course or curriculum and at the level of the unit of instruction or learning programme. Here computer-based intelligent tutoring systems have been shown to be effective through the provision of immediate response, specific feedback, opportunities for practice, greater cognitive engagements, individualised task selection and accelerated learning control (Hill 2015). This represents the future.

Today, faced with the challenge of individualising learning and the associated problems, the teacher can ignore the possibility of adaptive learning and simply address the needs of the body of students as a whole. This is the easy option but has serious disadvantages, as illustrated in the following example. An analysis of the examination results in a medical school showed that one-third of the class incorrectly answered questions on a specific topic. As a response to this finding, a decision was taken to restore a number of lectures on the topic which had previously been omitted from the curriculum. This may or may not address the performance problem with regard to the students who had given the wrong answers to the questions. It penalised, however, the two-thirds of the class who had mastered the subject and for whom the revised lecture course was not appropriate.

Here are a few things a teacher can do to introduce adaptive elements into the curriculum:

- Construct a course within the curriculum in such a way that students can move through the course at their own pace. If they complete the basic required modules ahead of time, they can choose in the time remaining to study the subject at a more advanced level or study other subjects.
- A range of learning opportunities can be provided within the curriculum enabling students to select those best suited to their personal needs. Students, for example, can choose to attend a lecture on a subject, view a podcast of the lecture, engage in collaborative problem-based learning with their peers, or work independently using an online learning programme. The extent and range of learning choices included in the menu for the students will depend on the time and resources available. A move in this direction is supported by the increasing availability of e-learning resources.
- Resources for independent learning can be adapted or prepared so that the students' learning experience is personalised to their individual needs. If students answer a question incorrectly in the learning programme, or if they indicate they are having difficulty understanding the question, additional feedback is provided immediately to address the problem. There is a lack of

evidence from the laboratory and controlled situations that supports incorporating learning styles into instructional design. Outside of the controlled environment, however, learning preferences and learning styles do matter. Learning preferences influence student motivation to take advantage of a particular learning opportunity and whether they use it or not (Tracey 2015). In our experience, students will choose to use a learning resource in different ways – working as individuals or in pairs, using the self-assessment section at the beginning or the end of the programme and using the audio commentary or text (Khogali et al. 2011).

- When learning experiences are scheduled in the programme, such as a session in a clinical skills unit using a simulator, the time allotted for an individual student is not fixed, but is dictated by the length of time necessary for the student to master the required skills. It is the standard that students achieve that is important and not the time spent learning.
- With the expansion of medical knowledge and the danger and problem of information overload, students can no longer study all aspects of medicine in depth. Time, however, can be scheduled in the learning programme when students do have an element of choice with regard to the subjects they study in depth to meet their individual needs. Up to a third of the curriculum time may be allocated for electives or student selected components (SSCs). This is discussed further in Chapter 20.
- Portfolios can be adopted as a learning and assessment tool. Students are encouraged to create their own learning programme and to demonstrate their learning in relation to the core and other areas they choose to study. This is described in Chapter 33.

It has been suggested that a school can be judged not on how it manages the average student but how it deals with the above-average student and the student in difficulty – how it smooths the pebbles and polishes the diamonds. With an adaptive learning programme personalised to the needs of the student each individual has the opportunity to be excellent.

Relevance

A major criticism of medical education has been a lack of relevance of the subjects taught, particularly in the early years of the medical course. This was highlighted in numerous reports on medical education published throughout the 20th century. Particular concern has been expressed about the teaching of the basic sciences, with a common criticism that the course content lacks relevance to the training of a doctor.

Pressures to critically examine the curriculum content and the relevance of what is covered include:

- The rapid expansion of medical knowledge and concerns about information overload, with knowledge doubling in the biomedical sciences every 18 months

- The development of new subjects such as genetics and telemedicine, which should be addressed
- The need to address important learning outcomes that have been previously ignored, such as communication skills, professionalism and evidence-based practice.
- If students understand the relevance of a topic to medicine and why they are addressing a topic they will be more motivated to learn. The demonstration of relevance creates a powerful and rich experience for the student. In general, students learn more rapidly if they are motivated and realise that what they learn will be useful to them in the future.
- Learning is more effective when the student is engaged in applying theory to practice. This requires the student to reflect and to think about why they are learning a subject, which in turn dramatically improves the effectiveness of their learning. Inert knowledge that is not applied remains only in the short-term memory.

With these pressures and the danger of 'information overload', it is incumbent on the teacher to question the relevance of his or her teaching programme. Relevance is an important consideration in curriculum planning, in the preparation of a teaching programme and in the creation of assessment tools for a number of reasons:

A focus on relevance does, however, create problems in curriculum design and implementation. It is important to guard against paying too little attention to the basic medical sciences and the understanding they bring to medical practice.

Relevance can be applied as a criterion to inform the difficult decision as to whether a topic or subject should be incorporated in the curriculum. Although what could be learned has dramatically increased and continues to increase, the time available in the curriculum remains constant. The problem for the teacher is what to include and what to leave out. A further difficulty arises from the fact that teachers in the early years of the curriculum may bring only the perspective of a basic scientist. They may not have practised as a doctor and may have difficulty in putting the topic into a clinical context.

Strategies to promote relevance in the teaching and learning include:

- A vertically integrated curriculum with clinical experiences introduced in the early years of the course and basic sciences addressed in the later years (Chapter 17). The BEME systematic review (Dornan et al. 2006) noted that clinical experience helped students to acquire a range of subject matter by making the learning more real and relevant.
- An approach where the curriculum and the students' learning is structured round clinical problems or presentations (Chapter 16). A set of clinical cases or presentations can be used as a framework for the curriculum and

this provides a scheme around which students, from the early years of their studies, can construct their learning in the basic and clinical sciences.

- The use of virtual patients online, where a student is presented with a patient whose problem relates to the subject they are studying (Chapter 27).
- Outcome-based education with a clear statement of expected exit learning outcomes and communication with the student as to how their learning experiences will contribute to their mastery of the learning outcomes (Chapter 8).
- Examinations designed to assess the student's knowledge and skills in the context of clinical practice. This can include MCQs where a short patient scenario is used as the stem in a basic science question paper, portfolio assessment and performance examinations, such as an OSCE.
- The use of new technologies such as simulators to provide the student with a more realistic learning experience where the application of basic science to clinical medicine is demonstrated.

It would be wrong to leave the reader with the thought that relevance is related only to the teaching and learning of the basic sciences. As discussed in Chapter 12 on the 'authentic' curriculum, issues of relevance apply to all aspects of the curriculum and need to feature prominently in decisions about teaching and learning and assessment programmes in undergraduate and postgraduate education.

Over to you

Reflect and react

1. Reflect on the use of feedback in your own teaching. Ask your students or trainees what they think of the feedback provided by you. By paying attention to feedback, you can promote a culture of positive improvement in your learners.
2. Look at your own teaching and assess the extent to which students are actively engaged in what they perceive as meaningful activities. Documentation in a logbook of the cases they have seen involves the students in an activity, but if the student does not understand the benefit of the exercise, it can be seen as a waste of time.
3. Individualisation and tailoring a learning programme to meet a student's individual needs offers many benefits but is difficult to achieve in practice. Can you adopt in your own teaching programme one or more of the suggestions in this chapter that would allow you to take into account the differing needs of your students or trainees?
4. Feedback, activity and individualisation are all key ingredients of a teaching programme, but if relevance is missing your teaching is unlikely to be successful. Do you pay sufficient attention to ensuring that students recognise the relevance of their learning experiences?

Explore further

Journal articles

Harden, R.M., Dunn, W.R., Murray, T.S., et al., 1979. Doctors accept a challenge: self-assessment exercises in continuing medical education. BMJ 2, 652–653.

Hattie, J., Timperley, H., 2007. The power of feedback. Rev. Educ. Res. 77, 81–112.
An important review of the educational uses of feedback.

Khogali, S.E.O., Davies, D.A., Donnan, P.T., et al., 2011. Integration of e-learning resources into a medical school curriculum. Med. Teach. 33 (4), 311–318.
A case study of blended learning where the students have choices as to how they learn.

Macqueen, D., Chignall, D.A., Dutton, G.J., et al., 1976. Biochemistry for medical students: a flexible student-oriented approach. Med. Educ. 10, 418–437.
A description of a biochemistry course that allows students to proceed at their own pace.

Guides

Dornan, T., Littlewood, S., Margolis, S.A., et al., 2006. How can experience in clinical and community settings contribute to early medical education? BEME Guide 6. Med. Teach. 28 (1), 3–18.

Harden, R.M., Laidlaw, J.M., 1992. Effective continuing education: the CRISIS criteria. AMEE Guide No. 4. Med. Educ. 26, 408–422.

Sandars, J., 2009. The use of reflection in medical education. AMEE Guide No. 44. Med. Teach. 31 (8), 685–695.

Taylor, D.C., Hamdy, H., 2013. Adult learning theories: implications for learning and teaching in medical education. AMEE Guide No. 83. Med. Teach. 35 (11), e1561–e1572.

Books

Clarke, J., 2013. Personalised Learning: Student-Designed Pathways to High School Graduation. Corwin Press, Thousand Oaks, CA.
The use of personalised learning in secondary schools.

Harden, R.M., Lilley, P., Patricio, M., 2016. The Definitive Guide to the OSCE. Elsevier, London.
A description of how feedback can be provided to a student.

Kaufman, D.M., 2010. Applying educational theory in practice. In: Cantillon, P., Wood, D. (Eds.), ABC of Learning and Teaching in Medicine, second ed. Wiley–Blackwell, Oxford (Chapter 1).
A short and helpful description of how to bridge the gap between education theory and practice.

Rogers, A., 2002. Teaching Adults, third ed. Open University Press, Maidenhead.
A classic text, which covers basic principles as well as providing useful hints for teachers.

Websites

Hill, P., 2015. Promising research results on specific forms of adaptive learning. <http://mfeldstein.com/promising-research-results-on-specific-forms-of-adaptive-learning-its/>.
A description of intelligent tutoring systems.

Tracey, R., 2015. Collateral damage. A blog by Ryan Tracey. <https://ryan2point0.wordpress.com/2015/08/04/collateral-damage/>.
An argument for not ignoring learner preferences.

SECTION 1

Being an enthusiastic and passionate teacher

The good teacher and trainer should have a passion for teaching and the ability to motivate the learner.

What is a passionate teacher?

The importance of a teacher having the technical skills necessary to teach students effectively and efficiently will be obvious to readers of this book – skills such as delivering a lecture, managing small group learning, or preparing an assessment exercise. Having only the technical skills, however, is not enough. Good teachers need to demonstrate a passion for their teaching if they are to motivate their students to learn. The passionate teacher conveys an enthusiasm for the subject and for their teaching. Student surveys have found that the 'master lecturer' not only presents the subject matter with clarity, but also conveys the content with enthusiasm and excitement. 'All effective teachers have a passion for the subject, a passion for their pupils, and a passionate belief that who they are and how they teach can make a difference to their pupils' lives, both in the moment of teaching and in the days, weeks, months and even years afterwards' (Day 2004). The late George Miller described the worst teachers not as those who knew less or taught less but rather as those who were uninterested in their students.

In his book *The Passionate Teacher* Fried (2001) argues: 'Only when teachers bring their passions about teaching and life into their daily work can they dispel the fog of passive compliance or active disinterest that surrounds so many students.' He goes on to distinguish passionate teaching from mere idiosyncrasies or foibles. These may make the teacher memorable for their students, but this is different from the passion we are describing. As Whitehead argued in his classic 1929 text *The Aims of Education*:

> *'The University imparts information, but it imparts it imaginatively ... A university which fails in this respect has no reason for existence. This atmosphere for excitement transforms knowledge. A fact is no longer a bare fact: it is invested with all its possibilities. It is no longer a burden on the memory: it is energizing as a poet of our dreams and as the architect of our purposes. Imagination is not to be divorced from the facts: it is a way of illuminating the facts.'*

Does it matter?

Does passion matter in teaching? The short answer is 'yes'. Effective teaching is the result of a combination of many factors but passion is at the heart of what good teaching is about. A teacher's passion and enthusiasm for their students' learning is important. Passion and enthusiasm are highlighted in studies of the skills and attributes of excellent teachers. The word 'passion' features regularly in students' descriptions of their best teachers – both the passion teachers have for their subject and the passion they have for sharing their knowledge and understanding with their students. In one study students were asked what makes an effective medical teacher. The two highest-ranking attributes selected by both senior and junior students were 'is passionate about teaching' and 'motivates and inspires the students' (Kua et al. 2006). A review of exemplary university teachers found that they enjoyed teaching, showed enthusiasm for their subject and made an earnest attempt to promote students' learning (Hativa et al. 2001). Bill Smoot (2010), in his interviews with 51 great teachers, found that each of them had an inner passion that drove them to excellence in their work as a teacher and also drove their students to excellence in their accomplishments. Passion in teaching is not a luxury or a frill that we can do without – it is the key element in students' learning. When the quality of students' learning is compared in different situations, the differentiating factor is frequently found to be the passion of the teacher – more than their knowledge of subject matter, more than the teaching strategy adopted and more than the learning technology incorporated.

Every teacher can be a passionate teacher

Anyone who has a love for their teaching can become a passionate teacher. Anyone who does not have a love for their teaching should not be a teacher. Passionate teaching is not found in teachers as commonly as one might hope. It does not, however, require exceptional ability. Fried argues that it is not just a personality trait that some people have and others do not have: it is something that can be discovered and learned. You may not be able to be taught how to be a passionate teacher, but you can learn how to be one.

Bringing passion to teaching is not easy – it is challenging but it can be done. Depending on your personality, your passion can emerge in different ways (see Figure 4.1). Teachers do not have to be extroverted or flamboyant in their presentations to be thought of as passionate about content. They can be reserved and refined in their delivery and still convince the learner of their enthusiasm and commitment to the subject and to the students.

Here are suggestions that may help; some are taken from the work of Fried (2001):

- In your teaching think about how you can share your enthusiasm for the subject with your students.
- Let your students see that you are working in partnership with them to support their learning and not just as an expert standing aloof.

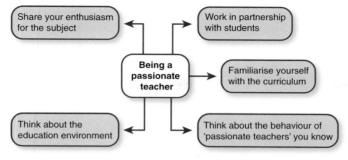

Figure 4.1 How to be a passionate teacher

- Demonstrate to your students that the course structure, the learning outcomes and education opportunities are clearly defined, and that the course examinations are fair and reflect the work of the course. Show that you are always looking at ways to make improvements.
- Create an appropriate learning environment that manifests interpersonal warmth, empathy, support for students' self-esteem, patience and a sense of humour.
- Care for and have a keen interest in the development of your students and feel responsible for their success and for their intellectual and moral wellbeing.
- Have a deep commitment to provide the best opportunities for each student based on their individual needs. Think about each of your students' potential and how you might build on their individual strengths.
- It helps to be enthusiastic about your teaching if you are familiar with the curriculum, how your own teaching fits in and why some topics are given more weight than others. This can help to guard against your passion for teaching being stifled or frustrated if you find that the time allocated for your subject has been reduced.
- Serving on a curriculum committee or course planning team gives you an added insight that you will find helpful.
- Think back to the teachers whom you most respected and learned from when you were a student. What was it about their teaching that inspired you?
- Think about the aspect of your work as a teacher that gives you the greatest satisfaction. Could you develop this further?
- Don't be surprised if you come across cynics who will try to dampen your enthusiasm. Expect to hear comments like 'You've only got a short time to teach on the subject so don't get carried away' or Your ideas will never work as there are too many students in the class' or 'We don't have enough resources for you to do that'. Keep in mind that most obstacles put in your way are surmountable.
- Think about bringing some of your passion outside medicine into your teaching. For example, I (RMH) have an interest in gardening and use it as a metaphor to illustrate educational principles.

- Finally, contact with others will sustain your desire to be a teacher. It may be with someone who has a similar passion for teaching, it may be through online communications and it may be through participation in conferences

Teacher stress and burn out

Teaching can be stressful for a number of reasons. Even the most enthusiastic teacher may be stressed, and over time can be subject to 'burn out'. This is associated with increased feelings of emotional exhaustion and fatigue, the development of negative cynical attitudes towards students and the tendency for teachers to evaluate themselves negatively, resulting in a feeling of lack of personal accomplishment. Teachers may at times feel overwhelmed with the challenges and workload facing them. A better understanding of their work as a teacher and how the different tasks faced can be tackled, as described in this book, may help the teacher to address the issues. If it remains a problem, assistance should be sought.

Over to you

Reflect and react

1. Recognise that much can be achieved by teachers who love to teach and by students who want to learn. Keep in mind that passion and enthusiasm, although difficult to measure, are a teacher's most valuable asset.
2. Remember that there is no place for teaching by humiliating and patronising students, but there is a place for teachers who demonstrate a passion for their teaching.
3. Are you considered by your students and colleagues to be a passionate teacher, filling them with enthusiasm for your subject? How do you convey your passion and enthusiasm to the students? Consider whether you could adopt some of the strategies outlined above to improve your teaching.
4. Are you fully committed to the performance of each student and to the extent to which they are achieving their individual potential? Do students perceive you as someone who is there to help and support them?

Explore further

Journal articles

Hativa, N., Barak, R., Simhi, E., 2001. Exemplary university teachers. Knowledge and beliefs regarding effective teaching dimensions and strategies. J. High. Educ. 72, 699–729.

A review of the attributes of effective teachers.

Kua, E.H., Voon, F., Hoon, C., et al., 2006. What makes an effective medical teacher? Perceptions of medical students. Med. Teach. 28, 738–741.

A survey demonstrating the importance of passion.

Books

Day, C., 2004. A Passion for Teaching. Routledge, London.

The importance of passion in teaching.

Fried, R.L., 2001. The Passionate Teacher: A Practical Guide. Beacon Press, Boston.

How a teacher can be passionate about their teaching.

Smoot, B., 2010. Conversations with Great Teachers. Indiana University Press, Bloomington & Indianapolis.
A description of how passion and enthusiasm contributes to great teaching.

Whitehead, A.N., 1929. The Aims of Education and Other Essays. The Free Press, New York.
A classic text.

Websites

Maintaining Passion for Teaching, 2015. <http://www.masters-education.com/maintaining-passion-for-teaching/>.

What stops a teacher being passionate about their teaching and how they can overcome the obstacles.

Villarroel, G., 2015. How Passion Can Make the Difference in the Classroom. Centre for Faculty Excellence, US Military Academy. <http://www.usma.edu/cfe/Literature/Villarroel_15.pdf>.
An interesting account of a study of passion in teachers at a military academy.

Teaching is both a craft and a science. Decisions taken by a teacher or trainer can be based on evidence of what works. Intuition and professional judgement also have a key part to play.

A 'PHOG' approach

Decisions in medical education about teaching and learning methods, about assessment approaches and about curriculum planning have been made in the past on what might be called a 'PHOG' approach based on the *prejudices* of the teacher, *hunches* of what works best, personal *opinion* and *guesses* as to the most suitable approach (Figure 5.1). Cees van der Vleuten, when he joined Maastricht Medical School, highlighted a paradox in medical education:

> *I noticed that my new colleagues – clinical and biomedical researchers – had the same academic values as I did which reassured me and made me feel comfortable. However I quickly noticed something peculiar; the academic attitudes of the researchers seemed to change when educational issues were discussed. Critical appraisal and scientific scrutiny were suddenly replaced by personal experiences and beliefs and sometimes by traditional values and dogmas.*

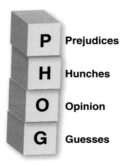

P Prejudices

H Hunches

O Opinion

G Guesses

Figure 5.1   The PHOG approach to teaching decisions

Since then, however, the need for evidence-informed teaching has been increasingly accepted, even if it has not been fully implemented in practice (Harden et al. 1999). A curriculum document from Maastricht, for example, describes the new Maastricht curriculum as an 'evidence-based curriculum'.

Evidence-informed teaching

It is accepted that an effective teacher, as highlighted in Chapter 2, requires a set of technical competencies, a basic understanding of education principles and a passion for teaching. But that is not the end of the matter – there is something else to consider. There is a need for the teacher to accept openly that there may be different and possibly more effective methods of teaching than those they are currently employing. They should not assume that the methods they experienced as a student or those in current use are the most appropriate, particularly at a time of change in healthcare delivery and in medical education.

In medicine, doctors are encouraged, as far as possible, to make decisions about the diagnosis and management of their patients on the basis of the evidence of what works and what does not work. This is the key principle of the evidence-based medicine (EBM) movement in health care. Evidence-based education – or more appropriate, evidence-informed education – has a similar objective. Teachers should make conscious, explicit and judicious use of evidence regarding what works and does not work in their teaching practice. This involves teachers integrating their individual expertise as a teacher with the best available external evidence. Teachers need to question whether a new approach advocated will prove better or worse than the traditional approach it would be replacing, or how their existing approach may be improved. The concept of evidence-based decision making was one of the three fundamental principles incorporated in the Carnegie 'Teachers for a New Era' initiative in the United States.

Evidence from research in medical education should be incorporated as seamlessly as possible into education programmes. Teachers, as suggested in Chapter 7, should document their own experiences and should make decisions about their teaching practice informed by education research. Research on what works best should be a routine part of medical education for those charged with formulating the vision or mission of the school, for curriculum and course planning committees and for the individual teacher.

Promoting evidence-informed discussions, suggests Goldacre, 'is not about telling teachers what to do. It is in fact quite the opposite. This is about empowering teachers to make independent evidence-informed decisions about what works by generating good quality evidence, and using it thoughtfully. The gains here are potentially huge' (Bad Science 2013).

Although there have been increased efforts to generate evidence about what works and why this is so, there has been less attention paid to the translation of evidence from research into teaching practice. Doctors have aids such as *Up-To-Date* to inform their clinical decisions. In contrast, there has been no equivalent source of information about evidence relating to education. This is a challenge currently being addressed by the Best Evidence Medical Education (BEME) Collaboration.

What is evidence?

What counts as evidence in education is a difficult question. Relevant evidence may come from very different sources, including professional experience and professional judgement as well as from formal experimental or quasi-experimental research studies. Evidence that can be used to inform your decisions as a teacher can come from:

- *Your own personal experience*. As a professional you should enquire into what works for you in your own setting and how the teaching and learning process can be improved (see Chapter 7).
- *The experience of colleagues*. A key factor in the introduction of the OSCE into medical schools in South Africa was the participation and experiences by teachers as external examiners in an OSCE in another school (Harden et al. 2015).
- *Experiences reported in the literature or presented at educational meetings*. Paul Worley described in *Medical Teacher* how eight students at Flinders Medical School in Australia received their clinical training in a rural community rather than in a teaching hospital and how they performed in the end-of-course assessment as well as, or better than, their colleagues. Despite the relatively small number of students studied, this provided useful evidence and encouragement for teachers interested in developing community-based teaching in their own school.
- *A published review, guide or editorial on a topic*. The Association for Medical Education in Europe (AMEE) Guide on Faculty Development by Michelle McLean and co-workers (2008), for example, provides a helpful summary of experiences with faculty development and how faculty development programmes are best delivered.
- *A systematic review of what has been published on the topic*. Systematic reviews, such as those published by the BEME Collaboration (http://www.BEMEcollaboration.org), use a systematic and transparent methodology and draw on the collective findings from primary research in specific topics to better inform education practice. Reviews look not only at the approach but why it works. The BEME systematic review on simulation, for example, identified ten features that improve learning if put into practice when high-fidelity simulators are used.

Searching for evidence

Searching for evidence to inform best practice in medical education is a complex undertaking if a thorough review of the literature is to be undertaken. BEME Guide No. 3 by Alex Haig and Marshall Dozier (2003) provides a comprehensive overview of relevant information sources. These include core bibliographic databases such as Medline, Embase, CINAHL (Cumulative Index to Nursing and Allied Health Literature), ERIC (The Education Resource Information Centre), BEI (The British Education Index) and PsycINFO; other less well known databases; and the grey literature, which includes print and electronic reports not commercially published, newsletters, theses and committee reports. The guide describes how to undertake a search and illustrates the process with a number of examples.

Evaluating evidence

Teachers often ask how published evidence can be evaluated with regard to its relevance in their context. The QUESTS criteria for the assessment of evidence (Harden et al. 1999) can assist them with this task. The criteria are as follows:

- **Quality of the evidence.** This relates to the type of evidence or research method and the rigour of the study. Qualitative methods have a place alongside quantitative approaches. The randomised controlled trial may in practice not yield the best evidence.
- **Utility of the evidence.** The utility is the extent to which the approach described in the research studies will need to be adapted for use in your own practice. Research on problem-based learning (PBL), for example, may be based on a small group size of eight students who meet formally as a group three times per week. The results and conclusions may have to be interpreted with caution if your group size is significantly larger and the meetings less frequent.
- **Extent of the evidence.** The number of studies reported and the size or extent of the individual studies are relevant. Evidence from a single case study that a new approach has worked well is helpful but it is useful to have this confirmed. There is a need for more replication studies in education.
- **Strength of the evidence.** It is important to distinguish between statistical significance and practical significance. Students in an experimental group may score 67.5% in the assessment and students in a control group 65.9%. While this may be statistically significant, it is of doubtful practical importance.
- **Target.** This relates to whether what has been assessed as the outcome in a research study matches your own expected outcomes. The evidence may be less relevant because the study addresses a different question from the one in which you are interested. You might be interested, for example, in the costs and logistics of implementing a new assessment procedure while the reported research has, as its aim, an evaluation of the effect of the assessment on the students' learning.
- **Setting or context for the study.** Geographical considerations or the phase of the curriculum may be important factors when interpreting any results. There is no such thing as context-free evidence and research findings need to be interpreted in relation to the context in which the research studies were conducted.

The value of reported evidence and the conclusions drawn from it can be considered as the sum of the power of the evidence (the quality, the extent and the strength) and the relevance of the evidence to your teaching practice (the utility, the target and the setting).

Best evidence medical education

Evidence-informed teaching is a philosophy that has two elements. First, it requires that a teacher should not assume that their current practice is optimal and no change is required. Second, the teacher should seek evidence that will inform their decisions as to the most effective teaching approach. There is a widely held view amongst clinicians, medical researchers and medical teachers that evidence to inform decisions relating to teaching is not available. This is not the case. For the most part, the recommendations in this book as they relate to educational strategies such as feedback, to teaching tools such as simulators, and to assessment methods such as the OSCE, are informed by evidence. Often those who are concerned about the lack of evidence have either not looked for it or have looked in the wrong places.

The BEME collaboration (http://www.BEMEcollaboration.org) was established with the aim of helping teachers make decisions about their teaching practice on the best evidence available. Systematic reviews of available evidence, produced on a wide range of topics, provide information about what works, in what circumstances and for whom. The reviews can help teachers to base their practice on available evidence.

The overall aim of the BEME Collaboration is the creation of a culture of evidence-informed decisions in medical education (Thistlethwaite and Hammick 2010). It has certain similarities to the Cochrane Collaboration in medicine (Patricio and Carneiro 2012).

The level of evidence available to inform decisions about day-to-day practice will vary. We are certainly not at the extreme right end of the evidence continuum shown in Figure 5.2, nor are we at the left end. As we learn more and more about what we do as teachers there will be a move towards the right. Best evidence medical education is now emerging from the shadows and becoming an accepted part of the delivery of an education programme.

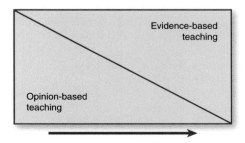

Figure 5.2 The evidence continuum in teaching

Judgement, intuition and teaching

It should be appreciated that the available evidence from research in medical education does not provide a dictat on precisely how to teach in a particular setting. Just as a doctor has to use his or her clinical judgement, so too does the teacher have to use judgement about his or her teaching. There may be no one answer about the best way to teach or assess the learner's achievements. The answer may depend on a particular context, subject, or student.

We return to our earlier assertion that medical education is both a science and an art. While an evidence-based approach to teaching is of value, intuition by teachers in their professional practice also has an important, although less well recognised, part to play. Teaching involves the performance of complex and diverse skills in real time and in contexts that are sometimes unpredictable and constantly evolving. Experienced teachers often cannot explain what they do and why they are doing it. This is not surprising as much of what a teacher does is intuitive – a reaction at the time to a situation and students' responses. Intuition can be thought of as the tacit knowledge built by the teacher out of accumulated information and experience. All teachers will need at times to use intuition when making decisions about their teaching practice.

Over to you

Reflect and react

1. Teaching is not simply the adoption of a 'cookbook of recipes' developed by others. Professional judgement and intuition needs to be combined with the understanding of the best evidence available so that the teacher can arrive at the correct decision and take the appropriate action. With regard to your teaching, consider where you are on the continuum between opinion-based and evidence-based approaches, as shown in Figure 5.2, and whether you might move further to the right.
2. Look at a BEME review, for example BEME review No. 4 on Simulation, and assess whether the conclusions have any relevance to your own teaching.
3. The next time you read an article, assess the implications of the evidence for your own practice in terms of the QUESTS criteria.

Explore further

Journal articles

Patricio, M., vaz Carneiro, A., 2012. Systematic reviews of evidence in medical education and clinical medicine: is the nature of evidence similar? Med. Teach. 34 (6), 474–482.
A comparison of the BEME and Cochrane Review processes.
Thistlethwaite, J., Hammick, M., 2010. The Best Evidence Medical Education (BEME) collaboration: into the next decade. Med. Teach. 32, 880–882.

Guides

Haig, A., Dozier, M., 2003. Systematic Searching for Evidence in Medical Education. BEME Guide No. 3. AMEE, Dundee.
Harden, R.M., Grant, J., Buckley, G., et al., 1999. Best Evidence Medical Education. BEME Guide No. 1. AMEE, Dundee.

A summary of the best evidence medical education concept and the factors influencing the need to move to evidence-based teaching.

Issenberg, S.B., McGaghie, W.C., Petrusa, E.R., 2004. Features and Uses of High-Fidelity Medical Simulations That Lead to Effective Learning. BEME Guide No. 4. AMEE, Dundee.

McLean, M., Cilliers, F., Van Wyk, J.M., 2008. Faculty development: yesterday, today and tomorrow. AMEE Guide No. 33. Med. Teach. 30, 555–584.

Frameworks for designing, implementing and evaluating faculty development programmes.

Books

Atkinson, T., Claxton, G., 2000. Intuitive Practitioner: On the Value of Not Always Knowing What One Is Doing. Open University Press, Maidenhead.

Harden, R.M., Lilley, P., Patricio, M., 2016. The Definitive Guide to the OSCE. Elsevier, London.

The objective structured clinical examination as a performance assessment.

Websites

<http://www.BEMEcollaboration.org>.

A useful collection of information about BEME and reviews and information about evidence-based teaching.

Bad Science, 2013. Teachers! What would evidence based practice look like? By Ben Goldacre. <http://www.badscience.net/2013/03heres-my-paper-on-evidence-and-teaching-for-the-education-minister/>.

The case for evidence-informed decisions in education.

Collaborating and working as a team 6

'*The quality of results often increases when a problem is addressed through collaborations.*'

Barbara Gray

Collaboration is important

In teaching, as in other areas of activity, we can achieve much more through collaboration and teamwork than we can do alone. If you look at any medical education journal you will see that few, if any, articles have a single author. Most have multiple authors with the work reported being the product of a team of contributors. The development and delivery of a course or curriculum, the design of a new learning or assessment strategy, and research into medical education, all require teamwork. In medical education there is the potential for a productive synergy between the different stakeholders leading to more effective, more efficient and innovative programmes. Collaboration may involve:

- the teachers or trainers responsible for a course or education programme, including the basic scientists and the clinicians
- students
- others in your institution, including education technologists, instructional designers, education psychologists, researchers and administrators
- other healthcare professionals, including nurses, pharmacists and physiotherapists
- other stakeholders, including patients, directors of hospitals and regulators
- those involved with the different phases of undergraduate, postgraduate and continuing education
- teachers responsible for the delivery of a similar education programme locally, nationally or internationally.

Collaboration has even been described as the lifeblood of the school or institution. A study in secondary schools in the United States found that students' achievements were greater when the teachers collaborated, when they had frequent conversations with their colleagues and when there was a feeling of closeness among teachers. These and other benefits could be achieved in medical education.

41

Collaboration between teachers within a medical school

Collaboration between teachers is essential for the effective and efficient development and implementation of the education programme. By collaborating, much more can be achieved with greater effectiveness, efficiency and time saved.

Since the 1970s, the need for collaboration to deliver the education programme in a medical school has been recognised more in some countries than others. It is now standard practice in most institutions for the design and implementation of the programme to be the responsibility of a curriculum committee and not to be left to individual departments or professors. Collaboration between the different disciplines and between the basic and clinical scientists is necessary if an integrated curriculum is to be delivered, as described in Chapter 17. Each member of the team brings to the collaboration not only their specific content knowledge and expertise, but also their individual teaching skills.

An atmosphere of collegiality amongst teachers is important and has been shown to contribute to student achievement. Teachers need to be supportive of and courteous and respectful towards each other, and demonstrate that they work together as members of a team.

Collaboration with others within your institution

Recent developments in education technology include e-learning, simulation, virtual patients and the education applications of social media. We also have a greater understanding of how students learn. For the full benefits to be realised, however, we require collaboration between teachers and education technologists, instructional designers, specialists in medical education and researchers. Experience has demonstrated that developments in medical education prove to be most successful where there is close collaboration between the content experts, medical educationists, technologists and administrators. Lack of such cooperation is one of the reasons why there has been a lack of progress made in areas such as curriculum mapping.

Collaboration between the different phases of medical education

In 1932 the New York Commission on Medical Education noted that 'Artificial segregation of the basic medical course, the internship, the training of the specialist, or the continuing education of the general practitioner is very likely to create serious gaps in the education of physicians which should be avoided.' In Australia, a Committee of Inquiry into Medical Education and Medical Workforce (1988) reported 'The Committee recognizes that, if it were given the task of designing a medical education system for Australia *de novo*, it might well choose to take quite different approaches. It would certainly wish to remove some of the discontinuities in the system.' More recently, in a call for reform of medical school and residency in the United States, Cooke, Irby and O'Brien noted that:

'There is no single agency responsible for regulating and financing medical education; multiple agencies participate in this process and often hold conflicting expectations of programs and learners. Each of the various entities has a vested interest in ensuring the highest quality of medical education, yet most work separately to promote innovation, and this lack of coordination sometimes has the opposite effect.'

Despite these pressures for change, much remains to be done if we are to achieve a seamless continuum of education across the training programme for a doctor.

If we were to design afresh a training programme for doctors, it is unlikely that we would end up with a programme divided into the separate compartments or silos of undergraduate, postgraduate and continuing education. Today we see attempts to bridge the gaps. In most cases the divide between the basic science teaching in the early years of an undergraduate curriculum and the clinical training in the later years has already been removed. The problems associated with the transition of medical students to clinical practice following graduation from medical school are recognised. Closer attention is now paid, as described in Section 2 of this book, to ensuring that students on graduation have the necessary practical competencies and that during the undergraduate programme they have direct experience of their future role through shadowing a junior doctor while a student. Short transition or bridging courses have also been found to be useful. The importance of lifelong learning and continuing professional development (CPD) is now also recognised and the ability of learners to take responsibility for their own learning is an expected outcome of the under-graduate programme.

Instead of separate curricula for basic medical education, postgraduate specialist training and CPD, we should have an extended curriculum starting when students are admitted to medical school and extending until they retire from medical practice.

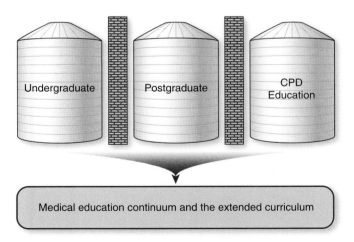

Figure 6.1 Continuum of education. The move from separate phases or silos of education to a seamless continuum with an extended curriculum across the phases

Lewis First, President of the National Board of Medical Examiners in the United States, argued at the AMEE 2012 Conference in Lyon that such a continuum of medical education across the different phases (see Figure 6.1) was highly desirable and could be achieved.

More generally, the concept of seamless learning connected across different settings, technologies and activities was identified in an Open University report in 2012 as an important development in pedagogy. As teachers, we need to support learners to develop their own system of learning across time and space. Portfolios can contribute to this, as discussed in Chapter 33.

Collaboration with other healthcare professionals

Teamwork and interprofessional collaboration is now recognised as a requirement for the delivery of effective patient care and patient safety. If we expect doctors to work as a team with other professionals once they are qualified, they need to be prepared for this as a student. Team and communication skills, and an understanding and respect for other healthcare professionals, should be reflected in the curriculum and the educational strategies adopted. Interprofessional education is now on the agenda in postgraduate education and in the early and later years of the undergraduate programme. This is explored further in Chapter 18.

Collaboration with other stakeholders

The planning and delivery of the education programme should be the responsibility not solely of the teachers in the medical school. A wide range of stakeholders should be engaged. As described by Vincent Dumez at the AMEE 2012 Conference in Lyon, patients can have important roles to play in defining the learning outcomes for the education programme, in planning the programme and in its delivery. Current students, recent graduates and the employers of doctors all have a role to play in curriculum development. Increasingly, curriculum committees represent these different interests.

Collaboration between teachers with the responsibility for a similar programme locally, nationally or internationally

At present it is expected that a medical school will take responsibility for the delivery of all aspects of the training programme. In business, outsourcing has become standard practice. One organisation might provide services for another organisation rather than it being provided in-house. In education, the benefits of collaborating with other institutions and outsourcing part of the education programme include cost savings, the opportunity to focus on core activities, quality improvement, access to additional experts and facilities and increased capacity for innovation. A medical school should no longer attempt to be self-sufficient in the delivery of the education programme.

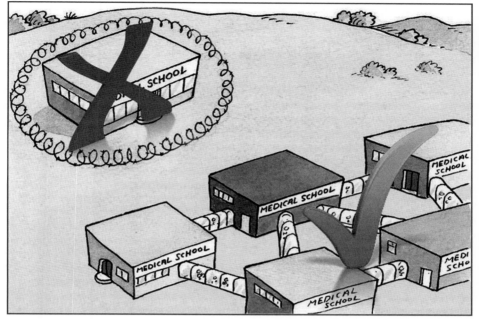

Figure 6.2 Medical schools should work no longer in isolation in the delivery of their education programme but should collaborate with other schools

The future will see greater sharing of curriculum planning, teachers, educational expertise, learning resources and learning opportunities (Figure 6.2).

Online programmes that cover some aspects of the medical curriculum are already available. This will increase significantly in the years ahead. The cardiovascular programme in Dundee (Khogali et al. 2011) had input from teachers in fourteen different schools around the world and students in Dundee had an online cardiology tutor located in Florida, thousands of miles from their own location.

Some institutions are now collaborating in the award of a joint degree. In their Prague Communiqué of 2001, European ministers of higher education called 'to step up the development of modules, courses and curricula offered in partnership by institutions from different countries and leading to a recognized and joint degree'. Recognising the international dimensions, we may see in the future the award of joint degrees in medicine.

Collaboration in practice

Why does collaboration not happen to a greater extent in education if the need for teamwork and collaboration in medical practice is now recognised? The answer to the question is represented by the formula:

Collaboration = (Vision × Shared Strategy)/Negative Mindset

45

The need for an agreed vision for the collaboration, a shared implemental strategy and the avoidance of a negative mindset are all important if successful collaboration is to be achieved. The book *Collaboration: What Makes It Work* reviews and summarises the research literature on factors that influence the success of collaboration (Mattessich et al. 2001). The need for an agreed vision for the collaboration with set limits is necessary, and polarisation should be avoided where some individuals are for and others against collaboration. This can be achieved if there is an imaginable, flexible, feasible, desirable, focused and communicable vision (Kotter 1996). For a successful collaboration there should be concrete, obtainable goals and objectives, a shared vision and a unique purpose.

A sharing strategy for the collaboration is also important, with good communication essential. The specification of learning outcomes in an outcome/competency-based approach to education as described in Section 2 is an important catalyst in this respect. The learning outcomes or competencies provide a shared language or vocabulary that is essential if there is to be an extended curriculum across the different phases of the education programme. This shared vocabulary also facilitates collaboration nationally and internationally and across the different healthcare professions. Internationalisation in medicine, with greater mobility of doctors and an emphasis on teamwork, are additional catalysts for a greater degree of collaboration in education.

Collaboration, however, is not always easy and may be hindered by a negative mindset against moving from the traditional model of teacher relationships to one where there is greater collaboration. There is concern that collaboration takes too much time, it destroys individual characteristics, it removes competitiveness and it generates personality conflict. There may also be a fragmented vision of the education programme with socially embedded knowledge structures within each group discouraging collaboration. On the other hand, John-Steiner (2000) suggested in *Creative Collaboration* that 'greater collaboration thrives on diversity of perspectives and on constructive dialogue between individuals negotiating their differences while creating their shared voice and vision'. At a time of financial constraints and at a time when there are increasing pressures for change, we may be forced to be more creative and to think about how we may collaborate in different ways. While some elements of collaboration are the responsibility of institutions, collaboration is also a responsibility of the individual teacher. Creating something better than we can achieve on our own can be satisfying and rewarding.

Over to you

Reflect and react

1. Could the education programme or part of the programme for which you are responsible benefit from greater collaboration with other teachers in your institution? Could other stakeholders, including patients, students and recent graduates, contribute to the development of your programme and its implementation?

2. Collaboration in the different forms and between the different players described has recognised advantages and can lead to more effective and efficient programmes and generate high levels of activity and innovation. Do you work with technologists, instructional designers and others to make your programme more effective and efficient?
3. Is there scope within your programme for introducing interprofessional education?
4. There is also a need for collaboration in education between teachers and others engaged in the educational programme locally, nationally and internationally. Might you usefully collaborate with teachers from other institutions, both nationally and internationally, in the development and implementation of your programme?

Explore further

Journal articles

Harden, R.M., 2006. International medical education and future directions: a global perspective. Acad. Med. 81 (12), S22–S29.
A move to greater collaboration internationally.

Khogali, S.E., Davies, D.A., Donnan, P.T., et al., 2011. Integration of e-learning resources into a medical school curriculum. Med. Teach. 33 (4), 311–318.
A case study of collaboration in the development and implementation of a blended learning programme.

Books

Cooke, M., Irby, D.M., O'Brien, B.C., 2010. Educating Physicians: A Call for Reform of Medical School and Residency. Jossey–Bass, San Francisco.
A critique of medical education in the United States.

John-Steiner, V., 2000. Creative Collaboration. Oxford University Press, Oxford.
An analysis of what motivates extended collaboration, coupling the effective and cognitive dimensions.

Kotter, J., 1996. Leading Change. Harvard Business Press, Boston.
A classic description of the process of change.

Mattessich, P.W., Murray-Close, M., Monsey, B.R., 2001. Collaboration: What makes it work? Second ed. Fieldstone Alliance, Saint Paul, MN.
An account of research into the nature of collaboration and what contributes to its success.

Reports

Committee of Inquiry into Medical Education and Medical Workforce, 1988. Australian Medical Education and Workforce into the 21st Century. Australian Government Publishing Service, Canberra.
A review of medical education in Australia

Final Report of the Commission on Medical Education, 1932. Office of the Director of Study, New York.
A review of medical education in the United States in the 1930s.

Websites

First, L., 2012. Achieving the continuum in medical education: who says it cannot be done? Plenary presentation, AMEE 2012, Lyon. <http://mededworld.org/Webinars/Webinar-Items/Achieving-the-Continuum-in-Medical-Education-Who.aspx>.
A plea for greater attention to be paid to ensuring there is a seamless continuum across the phases of education.

Dumez, V., 2012. The patient partner in care at the heart of medical education. Plenary presentation, AMEE 2012, Lyon. <http://www.mededworld.org/Webinars/Webinar-Items/AMEE-MEW-Webinar-76-The-patient-partner-in-care-a.aspx>.
A personal description of how patients can contribute to the development and implementation of an education programme.

*Teachers should take responsibility for their personal continuing
professional development and regularly assess and review their
own competence.*

Teaching as a professional activity

Teaching is a professional activity that requires:

- mastery of the subject matter that is being taught
- mastery of approaches to teaching that result in students' effective and
  efficient learning.

It should be apparent from the earlier chapters that teaching is an immensely
complex and multi-faceted activity that involves a wide range of competencies and
attributes, as illustrated in the three-circle model shown in Figure 7.1.

Teachers, if they are to meet their responsibilities, require a range of technical
skills that equip them to impart knowledge, teach practical skills, assess students,
conduct small group sessions and facilitate students' learning in a range of contexts. These technical skills represented by the inner circle in Figure 7.1 are covered
more fully in later chapters of the book. The teacher, however, is a professional

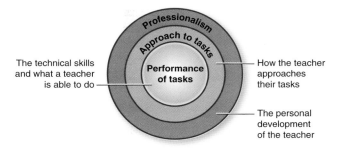

Figure 7.1   Three-circle model of the competencies required of a teacher

and not simply a technician. As described in the earlier chapters in this section, teachers have to approach their work with an understanding of the underpinning educational principles, with the necessary passion and appropriate attitudes, and using a combination of evidence-based decision making and intuition (the middle circle in Figure 7.1).

In this chapter we focus on the personal development and professionalism of a teacher. This is the outer circle in the figure.

Key professional responsibilities for teachers include the need to:

- reflect upon and be aware of their strengths and weaknesses as a teacher and be an enquirer into their own competence
- review current approaches and keep up to date with new approaches to teaching and learning.

Enquiring into your own competence

As professionals, teachers have to take responsibility for the quality of their teaching and for the assessment of their own competence. In choosing to read this book you have demonstrated your interest in teaching.

The expertise required to set appropriate standards for assessment procedures or to prepare an e-learning programme are obvious. In other areas, such as lecturing or the facilitation of learning in small groups, the expertise required may be less clear. Most teachers at some stage in their career will have given one or more lectures, run a small group session or counselled a student or trainee without necessarily having reflected on their performance in relation to the task. Assessing your own personal strengths and weaknesses is notoriously difficult. With students, for example, poorer performers are more likely to make an overinflated assessment of their competence. The same may be true for teachers. The teacher may believe that he or she has given an outstanding lecture, while in practice students find the lecture incomprehensible, boring and irrelevant. A teacher may use a small group session to express his or her own views and thoughts on a topic without appreciating that the students have not been engaged actively in discussion, nor have they been stimulated to reflect on their experience. A teacher may think that the counselling and feedback session provided for the students or trainees in difficulty has gone well, while the opposite is the case with the problem not addressed.

Here are some suggestions that may help teachers to assess their teaching prowess:

- Stop and reflect on your own performance as a teacher. By reading this book you have started this process.
- Study feedback from students about your performance. Students' views are obtained commonly through a questionnaire or a focused discussion. Feedback should address your coverage of the topic and your method of delivery and

presentation skills. Have you inspired the student to learn about the subject? The information obtained can be useful, but it has to be treated with an element of caution. In the classic example of what has been termed the 'Dr Fox Effect', a professional actor, unbeknown to the students, was briefed to give an entertaining lecture that was educationally poor. It was subsequently rated highly by students!

- Obtain feedback from colleagues. Peer evaluation of teaching is now standard practice in many medical schools. It is important that the feedback provided is constructive rather than destructive. Such feedback is easier to obtain if you are working as part of a team. If you know your peers well, you may be less inhibited to ask for their comments and more likely to trust their judgement and accept their feedback on your performance.
- Make a video of your teaching. This may be useful, and idiosyncrasies and defects in your teaching may become obvious. You can assess your performance on the video on your own or with a colleague.
- Take part in an Objective Structured Teaching Exercise (OSTE). OSTEs, which are modified Objective Structured Clinical Examinations (OSCEs), can be developed to help you assess your teaching skills in a practical context (Lu et al. 2014).
- Assess whether your students have achieved the expected learning outcomes. One measure of the effectiveness of your teaching is how well your students perform in written or clinical examination questions relating to the part of the training programme for which you are responsible. This information, however, may not be readily available to you.
- Assess whether you have influenced your student's or trainee's career choice and subsequent career. Such information may be achieved anecdotally from former students but it is a difficult outcome to assess.
- Study measurements of the educational environment in your institution. The educational environment can be assessed in your institution as described in Chapter 21. Your teaching may contribute to this.
- Participate in conferences on medical education. Participation in educational meetings or conferences provides you with the opportunity to compare your teaching practice with that of colleagues. By doing so you might improve your own teaching.

Keeping up to date

Medical education, just like medicine and health care delivery, is constantly changing. Over the past decade significant developments have taken place with curriculum planning including moves to outcome-based education and interprofessional education; with assessment including the wider use of portfolio assessment, work-based assessment and standard setting; and with new learning technologies including high-fidelity simulators, virtual patients and the use of the Internet.

Teachers in medicine have a responsibility to keep up to date not only with their subject area but also with developments and new approaches to education that may be relevant to their teaching practice. There are different ways of keeping up to date and we have listed some of them. You should choose the approach that works best for you.

- **Textbooks**. A growing number of books are available that cover, in more depth than is possible in this book, topics such as curriculum planning, teaching and learning methods, and assessment. A companion volume that discusses some aspects in more detail is *A Practical Guide for Medical Teachers*. If you have a particular responsibility in one area, such as organising an OSCE, you may find it helpful to read a text on the topic such as *The Definitive Guide to the OSCE*.
- **Journals**. Most teachers read the journals relating to their own specialty, but it is unlikely that the discipline-based journals will provide adequate coverage of medical education. Key international journals in the field of medical education are *Medical Teacher*, *Medical Education*, *Teaching and Learning in Medicine*, *Advances in Health Sciences Education* and *Academic Medicine*. Online journals such as MedEdPublish, BMC Medical Education and Medical Education Online also merit consideration. You may find more specialised education journals in your own area of teaching, such as *Education for Primary Care*, *Anatomical Sciences Education* or *Medical Science Education*.
- **Newsletters and online information**. Many professional organisations produce newsletters that help to keep their members up to date with education developments. Information on a range of education topics can be accessed using a search engine such as Google, through an online education community such as MedEdWorld (http://www.MedEdWorld.org) or by following an education blog.
- **Guides and reports**. The Association for Medical Education in Europe (AMEE) publishes a series of guides designed to inform the practising teacher about contemporary medical education practice (http://www.amee.org). Over 100 guides cover topics relating to curriculum planning, teaching and learning methods, assessment, management, research and theories in medical education. Systematic reviews of evidence relating to topics in medical education are published by the Best Evidence Medical Education (BEME) collaboration (http://www.bemecollaboration.org).
- **Conferences and meetings.** Attendance at a local, national or international conference or meeting where the theme is medical education is a popular way of keeping up to date. Some meetings such as the annual meeting of AMEE include in their programme workshops and master class sessions on a range of medical education topics.
- **Courses on medical education**. An increasing number of courses on medical education are available delivered face to face or at a distance. These may be of short duration or more extended and lead to an award of a certificate, diploma or master's degree in medical education. This book was written to support the online AMEE *Essential Skills in Medical Education* course.
- **Membership of professional education associations or communities of practice**. One way of keeping up to date is to join a professional organisation committed to medical education. This may be a regional educational organisation such as the Association for the Study of Medical Education

(ASME) in the UK, the Spanish Society for Medical Education (SEDEM) in Spain, the Netherlands Association for Medical Education (NVMO) in the Netherlands, or the Canadian Association for Medical Education (CAME) in Canada or an international organisation such as AMEE or the International Association of Medical Science Educators (IAMSE). Membership may include a subscription to a medical education journal, registration for conferences, and access to other membership services. It is worthwhile considering joining a network of medical educators such as MedEdWorld.org, which is an online global network of teachers in the healthcare professions who are committed to sharing ideas, resources and expertise in the field of medical education.

As a teacher you have a responsibility through one or more of these approaches to keep your teaching up to date, to know how your students can best learn, to recognise how the learning outcomes can be assessed and to understand how the educational activities can be organised into a meaningful programme or curriculum.

Scholarship in teaching

In his seminal work Boyer (1990) described teaching as one of the four categories of scholarship in a university. 'Priorities of the Professoriate' he argued 'is at the core of the university and teachers should be elevated (through the notion of scholarship) to a status equal to research.' Scholarship in teaching and learning requires teachers to:

- Reflect on their own teaching, noting what is successful and what does not work. 'The teacher is (or ought to be)' argued Martyn Hammersley (1993), 'a skilled practitioner, continually reflecting on her or his practice in terms of ideals and knowledge of local situations, and modifying practice in light of these reflections; rather than a technician merely applying scientifically produced curriculum programmes.'
- Share their experiences and communicate with colleagues within the discipline in their institution, across disciplines in their institution and regionally, nationally and internationally.
- Innovate and explore new approaches that work best in facilitating students' learning.

As a teacher you are a key player and a catalyst for change. You can help to change the world of medical education by understanding it and bring about change in your own context.

Over to you

Reflect and react

1. Reflect on how you obtain information with regard to your effectiveness as a teacher. Consider the different sources of information listed in this chapter. What are your strengths and weaknesses?

2. Think about how you keep up to date in your own discipline or field of interest. Can similar methods be adopted with regard to your responsibilities as a teacher?
3. Do you meet the criteria for scholarship in teaching as set out above?

Explore further

Journal articles

Hammersley, M., 1993. On the teacher as researcher. Educ. Action Res. 1 (3), 425–445.

A description of the teacher as an action researcher.

Lu, W.-H., Mylona, E., Lane, S., et al., 2014. Faculty development on professionalism and medical ethics: the design, development and implementation of Objective Structured Teaching Exercises (OSTEs). Med. Teach. 36 (10), 876–882.

Participation in an OSTE can help teachers to judge their own performance.

Vardi, I., 2011. The changing relationship between the Scholarship of Teaching (and Learning) and universities. Higher Educ. Res. Devel. 30 (1), 1–7.

An account of scholarship in teaching presented as an introduction to an issue of the journal devoted to this theme.

Guides

McGaghie, W.C., 2010. Scholarship, Publication and Career Advancement in Health Professions Education. AMEE Educational Guide No. 43. AMEE, Dundee.

McLean, M., Cilliers, F., van Wyk, J.M., 2010. Faculty Development: Yesterday, Today and Tomorrow. AMEE Educational Guide No. 33. AMEE, Dundee.

Books

Boyer, E.L., 1990. Scholarship Reconsidered: Priorities of the Professoriate. John Wiley and Sons, New York.

The classic text on the scholarship of teaching.

SECTION 2

What the Student Should Learn

'A good archer is known not by his arrows but by his aim.'

Thomas Fuller

- A key task for a teacher is to decide what the student should learn
- What the student should learn can be specified as learning outcomes, competencies and entrustable professional activities
- In outcome/competency-based education there is a switch of emphasis from the education process to the product and what the students will achieve
- Decisions about the curriculum, teaching and learning methods and assessment are informed by the expected learning outcomes and competencies.

The move to an outcome/ competency-based approach | 8

An important trend is the move from an emphasis on the process of teaching and learning to the product and what is achieved.

An important trend in medical education

The most important responsibility teachers have is to identify the learning outcomes or competencies expected of their students or trainees and to ensure that these can be achieved in the education programme.

Traditionally, medical education has focused on teaching methods such as the lecture and small group work, on the design of the curriculum and whether, for example, it was community-based or integrated, and on the assessment of the learner and the different approaches adopted. What has been described as the most important trend in medical education in the past decade is the move towards an outcome/competency-based approach where the emphasis is on the product of the learning rather than on the process.

The concept of outcome-based education (OBE) was promoted by Spady (1994). He defined OBE as 'a way of designing, developing, delivering and documenting instruction in terms of its intended goals and outcomes'. Spady suggested that 'Exit outcomes are a critical factor in designing the curriculum. You develop the curriculum from the outcomes you want students to demonstrate, rather than writing objectives for the curriculum you already have'. OBE can be summed up as 'results-orientated thinking'. This shift towards OBE is at least in part analogous to the total quality movement in business and manufacturing.

Outcome/competency-based education (OBE/CBE) is a performance-based approach at the cutting edge of curriculum development and offers a powerful way of changing and managing medical education. An outcome-based approach has been adopted by regulating and accrediting bodies such as the General Medical Council in the UK, the Accreditation Council for Graduate Medical Education in the United States and the Royal College of Physicians and Surgeons of Canada. Standardising of learning outcomes was one of the four key recommendations for programmatic reform of medical education advocated in the Carnegie review of medical education in the United States.

What is outcome/competency-based education?

OBE/CBE requires that:

- The learning outcomes/competencies expected at the end of training and at the end of each phase of training are clearly stated, explicit and communicated to all concerned including teachers, students and other stakeholders, such as employers in the health service.
- Decisions about the curriculum, including the content, the educational strategies, the teaching methods and the assessment are based on the agreed learning outcomes/competencies (Figure 8.1). These define what is taught, how it is taught and how it is assessed. They may even influence the selection of students for admission to medical studies.
- There is a collectively endorsed vision that reflects a commitment that students will succeed.
- The learners' achievement of the exit outcomes before they leave the programme of training is more important than the time spent in the programme. In OBE what is fixed is the outcomes or standards achieved with the time spent achieving these variable. In time-based training what is fixed is time and what is variable is the standard or outcomes achieved.

In this text we have not differentiated learning outcomes and outcome-based education from competencies and competence-based education. Although some workers have chosen to make a distinction, this serves no useful purpose and there is little value in doing so. The International Competency-Based Medical Education (ICBME) collaborators have been working since 2009 to provide an understanding of competency-based medical education and to accelerate its uptake worldwide.

CBE has been defined as 'an approach to preparing physicians for practice that is fundamentally orientated to graduate outcome abilities and organised around

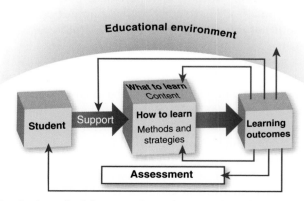

Figure 8.1 Curriculum decisions are based on the learning outcomes

competencies derived from an analysis of societal and patient needs. It de-emphasises time-based training and promises a greater accountability, flexibility, and learner-centeredness' (Frank et al. 2010). The idea of a competency-based programme in medicine was introduced by McGaghie et al. in 1978 but at that time had little impact in medical education.

Before we explore further the concept of OBE and how learning outcomes can be identified and grouped in domains within an overall framework we will look at the reasons why an outcome- or competency-based approach has now been widely adopted in medical education.

Why an outcome/competency-based approach?

While formal evidence for the effectiveness of OBE in medicine may be lacking, there are a number of strong reasons for the adoption of the approach. OBE offers major advantages, some of which are obvious, others are less so:

- **OBE highlights the competencies achieved by the learner.** What matters are the competencies and abilities achieved by doctors, including their knowledge, skills and attitudes, rather than how they were trained or how they acquired these competencies. This has been described as 'education for capability'. In the analogy of buying a car, the customer is more interested in how the car performs, its features and fuel consumption and how easily it can be maintained rather than details of the manufacturing process. As Thomas Fuller noted, 'A good archer is not known by his arrows but by his aim'.
- **OBE is necessary given the rapid advances in medicine.** Knowledge in the biomedical field is doubling every 18 months. For this reason it is no longer feasible to cover all aspects of a subject in the curriculum. While the amount of knowledge has greatly increased, the length of the undergraduate curriculum has remained the same at 4, 5 or 6 years' duration. It is now more important than ever that as teachers we agree and advise our students about the core competencies and knowledge we expect them to master in the time available.
- **OBE ensures consideration is given to important topics that otherwise might be neglected.** In the past there have been many areas that have been ignored in the curriculum resulting in gaps in the students' competence and errors in practice. Subjects neglected include attitudes and professionalism, communication skills, health promotion, team working, patient safety and management of errors. OBE helps to ensure that these areas are considered alongside other key topics.
- **OBE emphasises accountability and transparency in medical education.** Demands for greater accountability, quality assurance and transparency are features of medical education today. OBE focuses attention on standards achieved and not on time spent in training. An OBE approach to curriculum planning also encourages a debate regarding the aims of medical education and what is required of a 'good doctor'. This may include, in addition to the provision of quality care for individual patients, an element of social

responsibility or accountability in medicine and the development of the doctor as a global citizen (Hodges 2009).

- **OBE empowers students and points them in the right direction.** OBE provides a robust framework for the curriculum and can be thought of as the glue that holds the curriculum together. It is consistent with a move to a student-centred approach and provides students with a clearer idea of what is expected of them. Traditionally, when students embarked on their medical training it was more like a 'magical mystery tour'. They lacked an understanding of what was expected of them at the different stages of their education. The provision of a clear set of learning outcomes empowers the students and engages them more actively with the curriculum.

- **OBE provides the basis for the allocation of resources to providers.** The contribution made by a course or subject to the overall learning outcomes can help to determine the allocation of time and resources to individual courses. In one medical school it was proposed that the duration of obstetrics and gynaecology clerkship should be reduced significantly, given that the competence in the delivery of a baby was no longer an undergraduate requirement. The proposal was quashed when the contributions of the clerkship to the school's overall learning outcomes was considered. Among other things, the course offered students valuable opportunities at the antenatal clinics to understand health promotion and at the child and mother mortality conferences to appreciate clinical audit.

- **OBE ensures that the assessment is more valid.** OBE has particular significance for student assessment and the approach helps to ensure greater validity of the assessment. OBE is consistent with the move to a more performance-based assessment and facilitates an assessment-to-a-standard approach where it is the standards students achieve that are important and not the time they take to achieve them.

- **OBE provides continuity across the continuum of medical education.** A need to have a more seamless continuum between the different phases of undergraduate, postgraduate and continuing medical education is now accepted. OBE provides a standard language or vocabulary to plan the continuum and encourages continuity between the phases by making explicit the outcomes for each of the phases or stages of education. Learning outcomes provide a framework to anchor the education programme from admission to medical school throughout the lifetime of a doctor.

- **OBE flags up problems in the curriculum.** Increasing attention has been focused on curriculum evaluation. Learning outcomes provide a yardstick against which a curriculum can be judged. A failure to achieve the agreed outcomes almost certainly identifies a problem with the curriculum.

- **OBE helps teachers to select the appropriate topics to be taught in a teaching session.** The expected learning outcomes guide a teacher as to topics to be covered in a teaching session. They should not be tempted to cover the aspects of the subject that are only of interest to them. In the early seventeenth century, the practice at Glasgow University was for teachers to do just that. They selected a book from their personal or the university's collection that interested them and read it to students in the lecture hall. The senior university position of 'reader' exists even today although the role is very different. In response to student protests the concept of a planned 'curriculum' with the clarity of the content to be addressed was developed. This was the first use of the word 'curriculum'.

- **OBE facilitates mobility of doctors and enables curricula in different countries to be compared.** It is possible to compare education programmes using statements of learning outcomes. The Bologna process is concerned with harmonisation, not necessarily uniformity, in the higher education sector in Europe, and the Tuning Project has as its aim the establishment of a learning outcome framework for primary medical degree qualifications in Europe.

Myths and concerns about OBE

While OBE offers many advantages the approach has also been misunderstood and criticised by some teachers and educators. Here are some of the common myths.

Myth One: OBE is concerned with detail and the big picture may be missed

Concern has been expressed that what a doctor does is far greater than can be described in competence terms. In the 1960s Mager and others introduced the idea of instructional objectives. The approach, however, had a disappointing impact on student learning. A contributing factor was the level of detail in which instructional objectives were specified. The Southern Illinois Medical School had a book of objectives extending to 880 pages. Moreover, the classification of objectives into knowledge, skills and attitudes was inappropriate given the complexity of medical practice. These difficulties, however, do not exist with learning outcomes where the emphasis is on broader frameworks and the competencies required of a doctor. The three-circle or Scottish Doctor framework, as described in Chapter 10, demonstrates how outcomes can be designed to specify broadly what is expected of a good doctor.

Myth Two: OBE is a threat to the autonomy of the teacher and removes their freedom and independence

Concern has been expressed that defining education as a set of outcomes in advance imposes unnecessary constraints on the teacher. While this may be true in some fields, in medicine no one can disagree with the need for clarity as to what is expected from the doctor on completion of his or her training. Knowledge of the expected learning outcomes, far from limiting the role of the teacher, empowers teachers to devise their own programme to meet these outcomes.

Myth Three: OBE is contrary to trends in medical education

This concern was expressed particularly relating to problem-based learning (PBL) where a task for a PBL student group is to determine, in relation to a problem, their learning requirements. There is the need, however, within the context of PBL for students to be aware of how a study of the individual problem relates to the overall course outcomes. The move to OBE strongly supports a more student-centred approach to learning with what the student has to learn clearly identified, their progress based on their demonstrated achievement, their needs accommodated through different instructional strategies and each student provided time and assistance to realise their potential.

Myth Four: OBE is about minimum competence and excellence is ignored

There is concern that expressing the education programme in relation to what all students should achieve may set only minimum expectations and discourage higher achievements. As demonstrated at Brown Medical School, however, this need not be so with the student requirements set at three levels – Beginner, Intermediate and Advanced. Students have to achieve all outcomes at the Beginner level, some at the Intermediate level and at least a few at Advanced level. In a competency-based curriculum it is possible for students to move onto more advanced studies when they complete the programme at the basic level. This is explored further in Chapters 3 and 15 in the context of adaptive learning.

Myth Five: OBE is labour-intensive and the time required cannot be justified

The specification of learning outcomes and the implementation of an outcome-based curriculum does require time and effort. Much of this work, however, needs to be undertaken regardless of the educational strategy adopted. It is necessary if there is to be an authentic curriculum as described in Chapter 12. The benefits to be accrued, as highlighted in Box 8.1, significantly outweigh any disadvantages. OBE is not simply a passing fad and is now part of mainstream medical education.

Box 8.1 Features of outcomes-based education

Specifications of learning outcomes
- A broad framework of outcomes and competencies
- A vocabulary to facilitate collaboration in medical education
- Specification at different levels possible

A curriculum based on specified learning outcomes
- Freedom for teachers
- Empowerment for learners
- Time commitment rewarded
- A response to challenges facing medical education

Entrustable Professional Activities (EPAs)

What is an EPA?

Entrustable Professional Activities (EPAs), a concept introduced in 2005 by Olle ten Cate, have a role to play alongside learning outcomes and competencies in specifying what learners are expected to achieve.

Learning outcomes and competencies describe the attributes and the abilities of the student or doctor. An EPA is different. It represents a unit of work and can be defined as 'a unit of professional practice that can be entrusted to a sufficiently competent learner or professional' (ten Cate et al. 2015). The question asked in an EPA is whether the learner has the requisite competencies to carry out a specified task. Examples of EPAs reported in the literature include providing preoperative assessment, providing palliative care, managing common gastrointestinal infections and conducting a risk assessment (ten Cate et al. 2015). In the United States the Association of American Medical Colleges has suggested 13 EPAs relevant for undergraduate education (Appendix 1).

Granularity and EPAs

EPAs, as highlighted by ten Cate, may be small, e.g., measuring the blood pressure or taking a history from the patient, or large, e.g., carrying out a routine checkup of a stable adult patient or managing a clinical ward. There is an issue relating to the size or granularity of an EPA. The danger in specifying too many small EPAs is that this may result in the same fate as befell instructional objectives, where the large number of objectives became unmanageable and too difficult to apply in a practical context. The EPA should be sufficiently large, for example 'routine checkup of a stable adult', that it represents a significant step. Smaller EPAs (nested EPAs) may be combined to form a broader EPA (Figure 8.2).

Relationship between an EPA and learner outcomes and competencies

An EPA requires the learner to integrate multiple competencies from different domains. Each EPA requires a number of learning outcomes or competencies

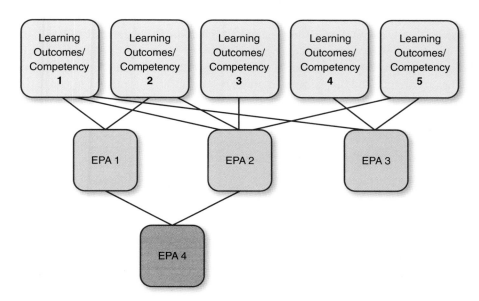

Figure 8.2 Each EPA requires a number of learning outcomes or competencies. Smaller EPAs may be nested in a broader EPA

(Figure 8.2). Combining together the learning outcomes from the different domains in a holistic approach to the patient is a feature of the three-circle or Scottish Doctor learning outcome framework described in Chapter 10. An EPA, for example, 'taking and recording a patient's history' requires mastery of outcomes from at least five domains in the three-circle model. These include domain-1 clinical skills; domain-2 communication skills; domain-7 information handling skills; domain-8 an understanding of clinical medicine; and domain-9 attitudes and professionalism. The relationship between EPAs and learning outcomes or competencies can be set out as a matrix.

EPAs and specification of the level of supervision

A feature of an EPA is that the level of supervision required at the given point in the training programme and against which the student will be assessed is specified. This may be classified as the ability to:

1. Perform under direct supervision with the supervisor present
2. Perform under indirect supervision with the supervisor not in the same room but immediately available
3. Perform with the supervisor available at a distance
4. Perform with no supervisor.

EPAs and the curriculum

Just as a curriculum can be designed round a series of learning outcomes or competencies, it also may be possible to design a curriculum around a set of EPAs. A comprehensive set of EPAs can contribute to the specification of the education programme. In this respect EPAs are similar to the tasks in task-based learning which, as described in Chapter 16, can serve as a curriculum framework. It is important to recognise, however, that a curriculum cannot be constructed simply in terms of EPAs. Some learning outcomes covered in a curriculum are not addressed in EPAs. For example, the development of the professional identity of a doctor, the ability to monitor personal performance and the ability to manage personal learning and to keep up to date.

Over to you

Reflect and react

1. Learning outcomes can help you in your role as a medical teacher. Think about which of the reasons described above for implementing an OBE approach are relevant to your own teaching.
2. Are there learning outcomes specified for the course or training programme for which you are responsible? If so, are you familiar with them?

Explore further

Journal articles

Aschenbrener, C.A., Ast, C., Kirch, D.G., 2015. Graduate medical education: its role in achieving a true medical education continuum. Acad. Med. 90, 1203–1209.

The contribution made by competency-based education to achieving a continuum of medical education.

Carraccio, C., Wolfsthal, S.D., Englander, R., et al., 2002. Shifting paradigms: from Flexner to competencies. Acad. Med. 77, 361–367.

An overview of competency-based education and the implementation challenge for teachers.

Englander, R., Cameron, T., Ballard, A.J., et al., 2013. Toward a common taxonomy of competency domains for the health professions and competencies for physicians. Acad. Med. 88, 1088–1094.

The development of a reference list of 58 competencies in eight domains for general physicians.

Englander, R., Frank, J.R., Carraccio, C., et al., 2016. Continuing to pursue a shared language for competency-based medical education. Med. Teach. In press.

A definition of terms used in competency-based education.

Frank, J.R., Mungroo, R., Ahmad, Y., et al., 2010. Toward a definition of competency-based education in medicine: a systematic review of published definitions. Med. Teach. 32, 631–637.

Griewatz, J., et al., 2016. Medical teachers' perception of the German NKLM professional roles – a multi-centre study. Med. Teach. In press.

In Germany, the National Competency-Based Learning Objectives were developed for undergraduate medical education and were agreed upon by the medical faculties.

Harden, R.M., 2002. Learning outcomes and instructional objectives: is there a difference? Med. Teach. 24, 151–155.

Hodges, B.D., 2009. Cracks and crevices. Globalisation discourse and medical education. Med. Teach. 31, 910–917.

ten Cate, O., Billett, S., 2014. Competency-based medical education: origins, perspectives and potentialities. Med. Educ. 48, 325–332.

A discussion between two workers in the field on competency-based professional training in medicine.

Guides

Harden, R.M., Crosby, J.R., Davis, M.H., 1999. Outcome-based education. AMEE Medical Education Guide No. 14 Part 1. An introduction to outcome-based education. Med. Teach. 21, 7–14.

A description and identification of the three-circle model for specifying learning outcomes.

ten Cate, O., Chen, H.C., Hoff, R.G., et al., 2015. Curriculum development for the workplace using Entrustable Professional Activities (EPAs). AMEE Guide No. 99. Med. Teach. 37 (11), 1–20.

A practical guide to EPAs and their use in the curriculum.

Reports

McGaghie, W.C., Sajid, A.W., Miller, G.E., et al., 1978. Competency-based curriculum development in medical education. World Health Organisation, Geneva. Public Health Paper 68.

An early conceptualisation of competency-based education.

Books

Boschee, F., Baron, M.A., 1993. Outcome-Based Education: Developing Programs through Strategic Planning. Technomic Publishing, Lancaster.

An overview of outcome-based education described as the supersonic jet model for the education of the next generation.

Hodges, B.D., Lingard, L., 2012. The Question of Competence. ILR Press, Ithaca, NY and London.

A thoughtful account of the concept of competency.

Spady, W.G., 1994. Outcome-Based Education: Critical Issues and Answers. The American Association of School Administrators, Arlington, VA.

A seminal work on outcome-based education.

Website

Greenberg, R., 2014. Core Entrustable Professional Activities for entering residency. <https://www.aamc.org/cepaer>.

Specifying the learning outcomes and competencies | 9

A range of approaches can be used to identify and define the expected learning outcomes.

Who is responsible?

The previous chapter highlighted the benefits to be gained from the adoption in education of an outcome/competency-based approach. The implementation of outcome-based education (OBE) is the responsibility of all of the stakeholders. The process of defining the learning outcomes required by the end of the training programme is often initiated at a national level. In the UK the General Medical Council has set out in *Tomorrow's Doctors* their expectations for the learning outcomes of a graduate in a UK medical school. There are similar initiatives by the regulatory or accrediting bodies in the United States, Canada, Australia, the Netherlands, Saudi Arabia and many other countries. National examinations where they exist may also be viewed indirectly as statements of the expected learning outcomes.

OBE and the specification of learning outcomes are now features of training programmes for many specialties in medicine, with the learning outcomes or competencies agreed by the relevant postgraduate training body or authority. In the United States the Accrediting Committee for Graduate Medical Education (ACGME) and in Canada the Royal College of Physicians and Surgeons have led the field.

While some learning outcomes are specific to the context of a country, there are learning outcomes relating to what constitutes a good doctor that can be shared across geographical borders. In Europe, through a consultation process, generic and subject-specific competencies expected of students at set points in the educational programme have been identified. The International Institute for Medical Education in New York defined in terms of learning outcomes what they considered to be the 'global minimum essential requirements' for a doctor, whether in China or the USA.

The specification of learning outcomes is both a top-down and a bottom-up activity. A medical school can build on a national statement of learning outcomes with an expanded version reflecting the particular mission of the school. A community-oriented medical school or a school with the aim of qualifying future researchers or leaders in medicine will reflect these orientations in its statement of learning outcomes. The Scottish medical schools, in 'The Scottish Doctor' report, specified the top-level learning outcome domains, e.g. clinical skills, subscribed to by all five Scottish schools. More detailed learning outcome statements varied from school to school, mirroring the differences in the curriculum of the five schools.

Within each institution, teachers are responsible for specifying the learning outcomes for each course and for each lecture or clinical training session within a course. These outcome statements identify how each specific learning experience contributes to the exit learning outcomes for the school's education programme.

For the most part, undergraduate, postgraduate and the continuing phases of education have been organised in separate silos, each specifying independently their learning outcomes and the design of their learning programme (Figure 9.1).

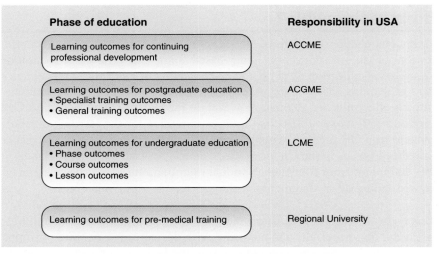

Figure 9.1 The learning outcomes and the different phases of education

Involvement of stakeholders

The specification of learning outcomes is a key step in the education process and the range of stakeholders should be involved. This may include:

- Specialists in the field
- Practising doctors in hospitals and in the community
- University teachers and educationists
- Students and recent graduates
- Other professions, e.g. nurses
- Representatives of employers
- Patients and representatives of patient groups
- The public.

The need for a wider consultation process is now accepted and is in keeping with a more patient-centred approach to care and a more general move to customer involvement in product development. Many of these stakeholders are now actively involved in curriculum committees. Such collaboration may help to align undergraduate, postgraduate and continuing education.

Approaches that can be adopted

The specified learning outcomes must match future expectations for the health care we want to see provided. Approaches that can be used to specify the expected learning outcomes include:

- Focus group discussions and a nominal group technique
- The Delphi technique
- A critical incident survey
- Studies of errors in practice
- Task analysis
- Interviews with recent graduates.
- A study of existing curricula and publications

Focus group and nominal group technique

Focus groups with representatives of the stakeholders can be organised to explore the specification of learning outcomes. This may be part of an iterative process. A nominal group method has been used to agree competencies and Entrustable Professional Activities (EPAs). This is helpful when some members of the group are more vocal than others and when there is concern about some members not participating. The procedure starts with a silent generation of ideas relating to the competencies and EPAs. Those are then shared and discussed. Finally there is agreement about the competencies to be adopted.

The Delphi technique

The Delphi technique is a commonly used and successful way of identifying the expected learning outcomes. It relies on the judgement of an expert panel of 'wise men'. The 'experts', usually about twenty although it may be more, are required to define the learning outcomes that they consider necessary for medical practice. The circulated responses are then analysed, amended and added to or deleted where necessary by the participants, and the process is repeated until a consensus about a final list of learning outcomes is reached. The Delphi approach has been used to identify learning outcomes for basic medical education and for training programmes in a range of medical specialties.

A critical incident survey

Qualified individuals (not necessarily doctors) are asked to describe medical incidents that happened to them or that they observed which reflected good or bad medical practice. As the number of individually described incidents increases, the incidents tend to fall into natural clusters and the areas of essential competence in medicine begin to emerge. Blum and Fitzpatrick (1965) described a classic example of the use of this approach by the American Board of Orthopedic Surgery. A variation of the critical incident survey is where those regarded as 'star performers' are studied and the features of a 'star performer' are identified.

Studies of errors in practice

Errors occurring in medical practice can serve as an indicator of problems with the existing curriculum, and identification of these can contribute to the development of learning outcomes. This may be carried out in collaboration with medical defence or medical insurance bodies. The identification of a common pattern of errors in medical practice attributed to poor communication skills provided evidence that skills in communication should have a greater emphasis in the specification of learning outcomes and in the curriculum.

Task analysis

Task analysis requires a researcher to follow a doctor on the job for a week or so and carefully list the tasks that the doctor carries out. The list provides a description of the activities that constitute the practice of medicine and can be the basis for the specification of the required learning outcomes. This approach is based on current practice and tells us what is done by a doctor today rather than what may be expected in the future. Nor does it give an indication of the competencies or abilities required to undertake the tasks recorded.

Interviews with recent graduates

Surveys of recent graduates can identify the strengths and weaknesses of the existing education programme and the stated learning outcomes. This can be done through interviews, focus groups or a questionnaire survey.

Study of existing curricula and publications

A useful starting-off point to determine the learning outcomes is to study what is currently taught in a range of medical schools or postgraduate programmes, and their related outcomes. Analysis of the content of current textbooks and other publications may also be helpful but should be considered alongside any changes that need to be made in the curriculum.

A mixed economy

None of the techniques described is a panacea for specifying learning outcomes. It is likely that the development of an appropriate set of learning outcomes will require the use of a combination of different methods.

Over to you

Reflect and react

1. If learning outcomes for your course have been produced, how were they derived and who was responsible?

2. If learning outcomes are not available, how would you set about producing them?

Explore further

Journal articles

Dunn, W.R., Hamilton, D.D., 1986. The critical incident technique – a brief guide. Med. Teach. 8, 207–215.

Dunn, W.R., Hamilton, D.D., Harden, R.M., 1985. Techniques of identifying competencies needed of doctors. Med. Teach. 7, 15–25.

Green, R.A., 2014. The Delphi technique in educational research. Sage Open 4, doi: 10.1177/2158244014529773.

Laidlaw, J.M., Harden, R.M., Morris, A.M., 1995. Needs assessment and the development of an educational programme on malignant melanoma for general practitioners. Med. Teach. 17, 79–87.

A description of how the learning needs were assessed for a continuing education programme for general practitioners.

Paterson, A., Hesketh, E.A., Macpherson, S.G., et al., 2004. Exit learning outcomes for the PRHO year: an evidence base for informed decisions. Med. Educ. 38, 67–80.

An example of the use of the Delphi process in the establishment of learning outcomes.

Books

Blum, J.M., Fitzpatrick, R., 1965. Critical Performance Requirements for Orthopedic Surgery: I. Method: II. Categories of performance. (AIR-56-2/65-TR). American Institutes for Research, Pittsburgh, PA.

An early description in orthopaedics of the application of the critical incident approach.

Jonassen, D., Tessmer, M., Hannum, W., 1999. Task Analysis Methods for Instructional Design. Lawrence Erlbaum Associates, Mahwah, NJ.

SPECIFYING THE LEARNING OUTCOMES AND COMPETENCIES

Describing and communicating the learning outcomes and competencies | 10

Different frameworks or models can be used to categorise and communicate learning outcomes.

Learning frameworks

Statements of learning outcomes and competencies are usually structured a round a number of domains – usually no more than twelve. Each domain represents a category of learning outcomes, for example clinical skills. Learning outcomes are then specified in more detail for each of the domains.

A number of frameworks or models for grouping learning outcomes have been described. Not surprisingly the different frameworks, while having significant differences, have much in common, with significant overlap between the competencies specified. Some of the most widely used frameworks are described below.

Criteria for a learning outcome framework

A learning outcome framework should meet the following criteria:

- The key domains identified should reflect the vision and mission of the institution as perceived by various stakeholders, including the public. They should reflect clearly, with an appropriate sense of values, what is expected of a doctor.
- The domains should be defined at an appropriate level of generality. The number of domains should be small enough to be manageable but large enough to distinguish different aspects of competence.
- The framework should provide a holistic and integrated view of medical practice and indicate the relationship between the different outcome domains.
- The framework should assist with the development of 'enabling' outcomes for each of the key domains specified.
- The framework should be clear and unambiguous. It should be intuitive and easy to use.

The Dundee three-circle outcome model and the 'Scottish Doctor' framework

This framework is based on twelve domains which are incorporated in a three-circle model. It differs from other frameworks as it emphasises the relationship between the different domains and shows how the different aspects of patient care do not function in isolation. The technical aspect of a doctor's performance cannot be seen in isolation. The aim for a doctor is to successfully integrate all the competencies (Figure 10.1). We have looked in Chapter 7 at a similar model for describing a good teacher.

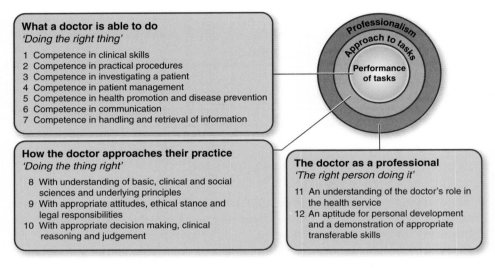

Figure 10.1 The three-circle model for learning outcomes incorporating twelve domains

The *inner circle* represents the technical skills of the doctor or what the doctor is able to do – 'doing the right thing'. It includes seven domains:

1. Clinical skills
2. Practical procedures
3. Patient investigations
4. Patient management
5. Health promotion and disease prevention
6. Communication
7. Information handling skills.

The *middle circle* represents the way the doctor approaches tasks in the inner circle – 'doing the thing right':

8. Understanding of social, basic and clinical sciences
9. Appropriate attitudes and ethical understanding
10. Decision making skills and clinical judgement.

The *outer circle* represents the development of the personal attributes of the individual – 'the right person doing it':

11. The role of the doctor
12. Personal development

This model is described in more detail in Appendix 2.

The three-circle model with the twelve outcome domains has been adopted in 'The Scottish Doctor' as a description of the abilities of medical graduates from the five Scottish medical schools. The approach has also been used in other countries.

The CanMEDS Physician Competency Framework

The Royal College of Physicians and Surgeons of Canada developed a framework built round seven physician roles. First introduced in 1996, this was revised in 2005 and again in 2015. The framework makes explicit the abilities of the highly skilled physician. The roles are:

1. Medical expert: Applying knowledge skills and attitudes to patient care
2. Communicator: Communicating effectively with patients, families, colleagues and other professionals
3. Collaborator: Working effectively within a healthcare team
4. Health advocate: Advancing the health and wellbeing of patients and populations
5. Leader: Participating effectively in the organisation of the healthcare system
6. Scholar: Committing to reflective learning as well as to the creation, dissemination and application of medical knowledge
7. Professional: Committing to ethical practice and high personal standard of behaviour.

Figure 10.2 illustrates the elements and the interconnections of the roles.

The CanMEDS competency framework has been used in postgraduate and continuing education in Canada and worldwide and has also been adopted for use in undergraduate education.

The Accreditation Council for Graduate Medical Education (ACGME)

The Accreditation Council for Graduate Medical Education in the United States developed a model based on six competency domains and thirty-six competencies closely aligned with healthcare quality aims. The competency domains are:

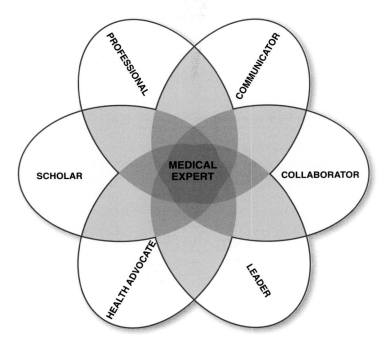

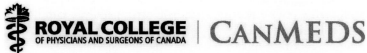

Figure 10.2 The CanMEDS Roles Framework
Modified from the CanMEDS Physician Competency Diagram with permission of the Royal College of Physicians and Surgeons of Canada. Copyright © 2015

1. Patient care   What you do
2. Medical knowledge   What you know
3. Professionalism   How you act
4. Interpersonal and communication skills   How you interact with others
5. Practice-based learning and improvement   How you get better
6. System-based practice   How you work within the system

The ACGME competencies are used both internationally and in US postgraduate medical education programmes to foster and assess resident physicians' development in the six domains. They have been adopted for the Maintenance of Certification (MOC) Program in the United States and are also used in undergraduate education.

The Brown Abilities

Brown University in the United States was one of the first medical schools to adopt an outcome-based approach to education based on a series of nine abilities. The

Brown description of learning outcomes is of interest in that it describes for each of the nine abilities observable behaviours that students must demonstrate at Beginning, Intermediate and Advanced levels of their training.

The nine abilities identified to describe a successful doctor are:

1. Effective communication
2. Basic clinical skills
3. Using basic science in the practice of medicine
4. Diagnosis, prevention and treatment
5. Lifelong learning
6. Professionalism
7. Community health promotion and advocacy
8. Moral reasoning and clinical ethics
9. Clinical decision making.

Global Minimum Essential Requirements (GMER)

The Institute for International Medical Education of the China Medical Board in New York, working with an international network of experts in medical education, developed as a set of learning outcomes the Global Minimum Essential Requirements (GMER). What is of particular significance is that they were designed from the outset around the competencies expected of graduates from medical schools in countries throughout the world.

The seven domains are:

1. Professional values, attitudes, behaviour and ethics
2. Scientific foundation of medicine
3. Clinical skills
4. Communication skills
5. Population health and health systems
6. Management of information
7. Critical thinking and research.

General Medical Council UK

The UK General Medical Council set out the expected outcomes for graduates from the UK medical schools in three domains:
1. The Doctor as a scholar and a scientist
   - Apply medical scientific principles to medical practice
   - Apply psychological principles to medical practice
   - Apply social science principles to medical practice
   - Apply to medical practice the principles, method and knowledge of population health and the improvement of health and health care
   - Apply scientific method and approaches to medical research

2. The Doctor as a practitioner
   - Be able to carry out a consultation with a patient
   - Diagnose and manage clinical presentations
   - Communicate effectively with patients and colleagues in a medical context
   - Provide immediate care in medical emergencies
   - Prescribe drugs safely, effectively and economically
   - Carry out practical procedures safely and effectively
   - Use information effectively in a medical context
3. The Doctor as a professional
   - Be able to behave according to ethical and legal principles
   - Reflect, learn and teach others
   - Learn and work effectively within a multiprofessional team
   - Protect patients and improve care

Over to you

Reflect and react

1. Agreement may already have been reached regarding the outcome framework that is used in your situation. If not, you can develop your own framework or select and adapt an existing framework. The latter approach has obvious advantages.
2. Are teachers and students familiar with the details of the framework and how the elements of the education programme for which you have a responsibility relate to the overall outcome framework?

Exploring further

Journal articles

2007. Med. Teach. 29 (7).

This issue of the journal has as its theme outcome-based education. It includes a series of articles describing the different OBE frameworks.

van der Lee, N., Fokkema, J.P.I., Westerman, M., et al., 2013. The CanMEDS framework: relevant but not quite the whole story. Med. Teach. 35, 949–955.

Zaini, R.G., Abdulrahman, K.A.B., Al-Khotani, A.A., et al., 2011. Saudi meds: a competence specification for Saudi medical graduates. Med. Teach. 33, 582–584.

Guides

Harden, R.M., Crosby, J.R., Davis, M.H., et al., 1999. AMEE Guide No. 14: Outcome based education Part 5 – from competency to meta-competency a model for the specification of learning outcomes. Med. Teach. 21, 546–552.

Reports

CanMEDS, 2015. In: Frank, J.R., Snell, L.S., Sherbino, J. (Eds.), Physician Competency Framework. Better standards. Better physicians. Better care. The Royal College of Physicians and Surgeons of Canada, Ottawa.

An introduction to the CanMEDS framework with a more detailed description of the CanMEDS roles.

General Medical Council, 2009. Tomorrow's Doctors. General Medical Council, London.

Scottish Deans' Medical Education Group, 2008. The Scottish Doctor. Learning Outcomes for the Medical Undergraduate in Scotland: A Foundation for Competent and Reflective Practitioners. Association for

Medical Education in Europe (AMEE), Dundee.

A description of the 12 outcome domains sub-divided into a more detailed set of learning outcomes.

Websites

Australian Curriculum Revision Working Group. Australian Curriculum Framework for Junior Doctors. <http://curriculum.cpmec.org.au>.

Brown University, 2015. Evaluation and Assessment: The Nine Abilities. <http://www.brown.edu/academics/medical/education/evaluation-and-assessment>.

DESCRIBING AND COMMUNICATING THE LEARNING OUTCOMES AND COMPETENCIES

Implementing an outcome-based approach in practice **11**

Outcome-based education requires two things. The learning outcomes need to be identified and specified. Decisions about the curriculum must be based on the specific outcomes.

The ostriches, the peacocks and the beavers

Outcome-based education (OBE), as discussed in Chapter 8, involves more than simply defining and publishing a set of learning outcomes that must be achieved before the end of the course. OBE is characterised by a curriculum where the learning strategies and learning opportunities are designed to ensure that students achieve the learning outcomes specified and where the assessment process matches the learning outcomes. Remediation and enrichment for students is provided as appropriate.

Despite a recognition of the importance of OBE, implementation in practice is challenging and teachers have not found it easy to incorporate OBE into their curriculum. Some principles, such as a move from a time-based model to an outcome-based model, are difficult to put into practice. Some learning outcomes, such as professionalism, are more difficult to incorporate into the curriculum.

Teachers react differently when it comes to implementing OBE. Harden (2007a) used the analogy of ostriches, peacocks and beavers. Some teachers consider OBE to be a passing fad and have made no effort either to prepare learning outcomes or to incorporate them into their teaching. They have buried their heads in the sand and can be likened to ostriches. Then there are teachers who work hard producing a set or list of learning outcomes that is prominently displayed for visitors or programme assessors – the peacocks. Unfortunately they do not adopt an outcome-based approach in their teaching, so their efforts are to no avail. The teachers who do successfully implement an OBE approach are those who believe that it is the way to design, deliver and document instruction. They work hard to make this happen – the beavers.

Implementing an OBE programme

An OBE curriculum starts with the question – what expected learning outcomes are to be achieved by the end of the programme and what capabilities should the graduate have as a practising doctor? An outcome framework is used, as described in Chapter 10, to describe the broad performance capabilities. These are each then specified in more detail. For example, in the broad domain of patient management a more detailed set of learning outcomes includes surgery, drugs, physiotherapy, social interventions and alternative therapies.

After the exit learning outcomes are defined, working backwards, outcomes are specified for each of the courses or attachments in the curriculum. These will identify how the course contributes to the school's learning outcomes. For example, the learning outcomes achieved in an anatomy course may go beyond the mastery and understanding of anatomy and, as identified by Pawlina in the Mayo Clinic, can include communication skills and teamwork. The outcomes are specified further for each of the learning experiences in a course or attachment, for example a lecture, a clinical session or a practical experience. It is helpful to produce a grid or blueprint that relates each of the learning experiences to the learning outcomes for the course. A similar grid should be produced that relates the assessment to the learning outcomes. The clearer the definition of learning outcomes, the more effectively student assessment can be planned. The appropriate tools are selected according to the outcomes to be assessed. An assessment profile can be produced for each student that highlights the outcomes that have and those that have not been achieved.

Student progression in an OBE curriculum

Milestones may be specified for each stage of the education programme. These are defined observable indicators of the individual's progress for their development. It is recognised that there are legitimate differences in the manner and rate at which students reach these milestones and progress to the exit learning outcomes. Some students, for example, may acquire the necessary communication skills more quickly than others. Students' achievements of the learning outcomes can be used to monitor and plan for their progression through the curriculum. Mastery of an outcome to a specified standard may be a requirement before the student is allowed to progress from one part of the medical course to the next. A student may be required, for example, to have a certain mastery not only of basic sciences but of communication skills before proceeding to clinical studies in the later years of the course. Progression can also be charted across the continuum of education from undergraduate through postgraduate to continuing education. A learner's progression is discussed further in Chapter 14.

Implementation guidelines

Outcome-based education may be associated with fundamental changes in the curriculum, for example with a move from a time-based to an outcome-based model or, at the less ambitious end of the spectrum, specified learning outcomes are simply embedded into an existing curriculum. The following guidelines may assist with the challenging task of implementing OBE in the curriculum.

1. The introduction of a competency-based approach in a time-based system while difficult is possible. This was illustrated in the orthopaedic programme

at the University of Toronto. Graduates have to demonstrate competency rather than spend a set amount of time in training. Easier to implement is a hybrid approach where there are elements of a competency-based approach in a time-based system. For example:

- Adjust the time students spend in a learning situation such as a clinical skills laboratory using simulators based on their mastery of the learning outcomes, e.g. auscultation of the chest, and not the time spent there.
- Once students have achieved the required learning outcomes for the course, offer them the opportunity for further study which may count towards their later training.

2. Ensure that staff are familiar with and receptive to the introduction of an outcome-based approach.
   - Staff may be unfamiliar with the approach and a staff development programme is essential.
   - Demonstrate to staff and students the advantages of implementing an outcome-based approach.
   - Discuss with staff what they expect of a graduate of the school.
   - Empower staff by giving them some responsibility and autonomy within the programme.
   - Encourage staff to work as members of a team.

3. Ensure that the culture of the institution reflects the move to an outcome-based approach.
   - The move to an outcome-based approach should be reflected in the school's mission statement.
   - The Dean and other senior figures should endorse and support the move.
   - Students should be supported in achieving the learning outcomes.

4. Prepare a curriculum map that includes the learning outcomes.
   - The curriculum blueprint should relate the learning outcomes to the learning experience and to the assessment.

5. Pay particular attention to outcomes that are more difficult to address, such as professionalism.
   - Be creative in your teaching approach, e.g. arrange for students to shadow a junior doctor and to discuss with the doctor the learning outcome.
   - Address the learning outcome across the undergraduate, postgraduate and continuing education phases of the curriculum.

6. Encourage a scholarly approach.
   - Undertake research to demonstrate the success of the programme.
   - Communicate your experience with colleagues at conferences and through other channels.

An OBE implementation inventory

An OBE implementation inventory can be used to describe a school's or postgraduate body's level of adoption of an OBE approach in their education programme. This can be rated on a five-point scale in each of nine dimensions, as shown in Figure 11.1:

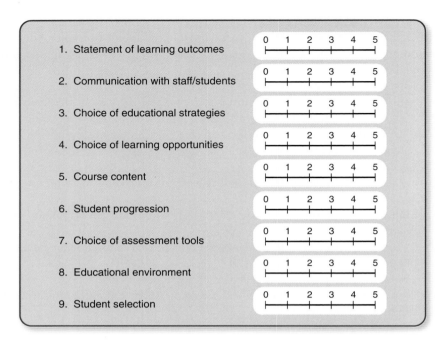

Figure 11.1 OBE implementation inventory

1. The extent to which there is a clear and unambiguous statement of the learning outcomes expected.
2. Whether staff and students in an institution are aware of and are familiar with the outcome statements.
3. The extent to which educational strategies adopted for the curriculum, such as problem-based learning, community-based learning or interprofessional learning, reflect the learning outcomes.
4. The matching of the learning opportunities provided with the learning outcomes. Almost certainly this will require the use of a range of teaching and learning methods.
5. Decision about content to be included based on the learning outcomes.
6. Assessment of students' progression through the curriculum based on their achievement of the learning outcomes.
7. Assessment procedures matched to the learning outcomes. Serious problems arise when there is a mismatch between the learning outcomes, the learning experience and the student assessment.
8. The educational environment (see Chapter 21) reflects the learning outcomes. A learning outcome addressing teamwork skills, for example, suggests the need for an educational environment that supports collaborative working rather than the more typical environment where competition is rewarded.
9. Reflection of the learning outcomes in the selection process for the admission of students to the medical school. Students can be assessed on entry-level requirements for each of the outcome domains, such as communication skills, problem solving and attitudes.

Over to you

Reflect and react

1. Where on the OBE inventory does your school or postgraduate body lie? Are you well on the way to an outcome-based approach or are you still at the early stages of implementation?
2. Have you clearly identified outcomes for your own areas of teaching responsibility and is it clear how these contribute to the overall outcomes for the training or education programme?
3. Consider how you use learning outcomes to monitor and guide students' progression.

Explore further

Journal articles

Dath, D., Iobst, W., 2010. The importance of faculty development in the transition to competency-based medical education. Med. Teach. 32, 683–686.

Harden, R.M., 2007a. Outcome-based education – the ostrich, the peacock and the beaver. Med. Teach. 29, 666–671.

A description of the OBE implementation inventory and how it helps teachers, schools and education bodies to create a profile of the extent to which OBE has been implemented in the institution.

Harden, R.M., 2007b. Learning outcomes as a tool to assess progression. Med. Teach. 29, 678–682.

A description of how students progress to the achievement of learning outcomes.

Holmboe, E.S., Ward, D.S., Reznick, R.K., et al., 2011. Faculty development in assessment: the missing link in competency-based medical education. Acad. Med. 86, 460–467.

The authors argue that medical education needs an international initiative of faculty development around competency-based medical education.

Sklar, D.P., 2015. Competencies, milestones and entrustable professional activities: what they are, what they could be. Acad. Med. 90, 395–397.

Turner, S.R., White, J.S., Poth, C., et al., 2012. Learning the CanMEDS roles in a near-peer shadowing program: a mixed methods randomized control trial. Med. Teach. 34, 888–892.

A description of the application of CanMEDS roles in practice.

Website

Fain, P., 2014. Competencies come to campus. <https://www.insidehighered.com/news/2014/04/22/new-competency-based-programs-lipscomb-could-be-model-liberal-arts-colleges>.

SECTION 3

Curriculum Development

'Teachers don't merely deliver the curriculum. They develop, define it and interpret it too.'

Michael Fullan and Andrew Hargreaves. *Understanding Teacher Development*, 1994

- Planning and implementing an authentic curriculum that meets today's needs presents a significant challenge
- The curriculum is more than just a syllabus or timetable. It embraces all of the learning opportunities for students, both formal and informal
- The ten questions described provide a useful checklist for planning and evaluating a curriculum
- Sequencing the content can prove complex. Some approaches may be more effective than others in helping the learner achieve the expected learning outcomes
- Students should be partners in curriculum development and not just consumers. The role of the teacher has to change as we empower students to take more responsibility for their own learning
- A clinical problem or task undertaken by a healthcare professional can serve as the basis for learning. The student is motivated by the more authentic learning experience
- An integrated curriculum, bringing together different disciplines, offers major advantages
- There are benefits from sharing learning experiences with different professions
- There is no better way to learn than from work-related experience. This requires careful monitoring and supervision
- Alongside a core curriculum that provides the necessary breadth of study, options and electives provide an opportunity for students to study selected topics in depth
- The education environment is now recognized as being a substantial and very real element that influences students' learning. Tools are available to assess the education environment
- A clear picture of how learning outcomes, teaching methods and student assessment link together is crucial not only for the teacher but also for the student. A curriculum map is needed.

The 'authentic' curriculum **12**

The curriculum is more than just a syllabus or timetable. It embraces all of the learning opportunities both formal and informal.

The concept of a curriculum

The curriculum was equated in the past with the syllabus and the timetable for the education programme. A curriculum document included a statement about content, the subjects covered and the courses that students should attend. This concept of a curriculum has been widened to include:

- the learning outcomes
- the teaching and learning methods
- the educational strategies
- the context for the learning
- the learning environment
- the assessment procedures.

Each of these aspects of a curriculum is explored in more detail in the chapters that follow. A curriculum can be thought of as made up of all the experiences learners have that enable them to achieve the specified learning outcomes (Grant 2014).

The curriculum is seen as an expression of intentions, mechanisms and context of the education programme that requires input from all of the stakeholders, including teachers, students, administrators, employers, the government and the wider public.

The 'authentic' curriculum – from university to the real world

In medical education we see a move to what has been described as an 'authentic curriculum'. Indeed this is at the very heart of medical education today. An authentic curriculum has as its aim that the learners will have the ability to perform in the workplace as an outcome of the education programme. Medical schools have been criticised and are being pressed to ensure that the doctors trained are able to meet the healthcare needs of the population that they serve. In line with the concept of an 'authentic curriculum' is a move to:

- an outcome-based approach, as described in Section 1 of this book, with an emphasis on professionalism, empathy, self-regulation and cultural sensitivity
- education strategies such as integration, interprofessional education, problem-based and task-based learning
- a socially accountable medical school.

In the authentic curriculum what is learned in medical school focuses on and connects with real-world issues, problems and applications. Unlike the situation in a traditional curriculum where the emphasis is on acquiring knowledge and skills to pass an examination, in an authentic curriculum students acquire the foundational skills, knowledge, understanding and attitudes that they will need to practise as a doctor. This involves 'connectedness', where the teaching has value and meaning in the real world.

In the traditional apprenticeship model in medicine, which existed for hundreds of years, knowledge and skills were passed down from one person to another. The apprentice learned from the master by observing him treat patients. Early in the 20th century, 'real-world' learning experiences that were a feature of the apprenticeship model were replaced in many countries by an emphasis on the medical sciences. This had the unintended consequence of separating the basic medical sciences and clinical practice. The fact that basic science knowledge should have a clinical purpose and not be an objective in itself was ignored in medical training until later in the 20th century.

Relevance as described in the FAIR principles (see Chapter 3) is key to effective learning. Studies have demonstrated that students' engagement with their studies is directly related to their perception of the relevance of the content. As illustrated in Figure 12.1, relevance can be seen as relating to the intrinsic value of what is taught, for example knowledge of hormone synthesis pathway in the thyroid gland will help the student to understand the actions of antithyroid drugs in the treatment of a patient with thyrotoxicosis. The other aspect of relevance is the 'instrumental value'. This is a demonstration of the relevance where the content is shown to be immediately useful in practice. Four quadrants are shown in the figure. The bottom left quadrant can be identified as the 'Ivory Tower', where there is no intrinsic or instrumental value of what is being taught. This sadly remains the home of much of what is covered in the medical curriculum. In the bottom right quadrant students have the opportunity to apply what they have learned but it is not relevant to medical practice. This is typical of many practical classes. For this reason many practical classes in medical education have now been replaced with more meaningful learning experiences. In the top left quadrant we have superficial authenticity. Here the teaching is dressed up to appear authentic by reference to real-world elements. This may be simply tokenism and such camouflage is not authenticity. It is not sufficient simply to tell the students that what they are learning has applications in medicine. They must appreciate this in practice through patients they see, 'Making narrow

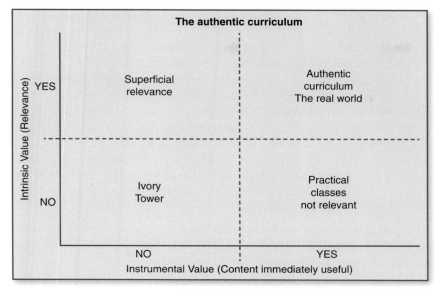

Figure 12.1 The authentic curriculum

pitches to a subject's future utility typically fails to generate student interest' (Cooper 2014). In the top right quadrant we have the authentic curriculum in the real world. 'Authentic academic tasks', argue Krajcik and Blumenfeld (2006), 'ask students to engage with content as though they were practitioners in that field. Such authentic learning is vital if students are to acquire the competencies necessary to practise as a doctor. There is no substitute for learning knowledge and skills in contexts that reflect the way the knowledge will be useful in "real life".' Bleakley and Bligh (2008) made an appeal for medical education 'to get real and engage students and patients in collaborative knowledge production, where real patients represent students' texts'. Central to their argument is that work-based learning should be the focus of curriculum design in medicine.

There are four features of authentic learning as described by Rule (2006):
1. The activity involves real-world problems
2. Students are emotional stakeholders in the problems and exercise higher levels of thinking as they learn
3. Authentic learning occurs through discourse among a community of learners
4. Learning is student-centred and students are empowered to direct their own learning.

The introduction of an authentic curriculum particularly in the early years is not without problems:

- The student may find it difficult to integrate the required knowledge and skills obtained from multiple sources

- The results are not always predictable and there may be unintended consequences
- The learning may be perceived as being inefficient
- Students may feel uncomfortable and even incompetent
- Teachers may not have the relevant background and clinical experience.

With thought and consideration, however, it is possible to change from a more traditional to an 'authentic curriculum'. Returning to the concept of apprenticeship, Dornan (2005) has suggested that apprenticeship is as relevant today as it was a century ago, 'I suggest the wheel has come full circle. Apprenticeship, central to Osler and Flexner's educational visions, needs to be revitalized ... The challenge is not to create a new educational theory, but to re-apply an old one to the fast-changing context of the 21st century healthcare.'

The planned, the delivered and the learned curriculum

A distinction can be made between:

- the *'planned' curriculum* that is documented and agreed by the curriculum planners and teachers and embodies their intentions and aspirations – the curriculum on paper
- the *'actual' or 'delivered' curriculum*, which is the reality of the students' or trainees' experiences and is what is delivered or happens in practice – the curriculum in action
- the *'learned curriculum'*, which represents the students' knowledge, skills and attitudes that result from their learning experience.

A mismatch between the 'planned' and the 'delivered' curriculum may be due to a teacher's lack of familiarity or acceptance of the specified curriculum, or to the fact that the realities of any course will never fully match the hopes and intentions of the planners. Occasionally the problem may arise from a deliberate intent by teachers to emphasise what they think is important to be taught rather than what is specified in the curriculum. Teachers can sabotage a curriculum. They need to be committed to the planned curriculum and accept the underlying principles. It is the teacher's responsibility to keep any differences between the planned and delivered curriculum to a minimum. Where there are significant differences, the reason for these should be analysed and action taken as necessary. Logistical problems, problems with students or trainees or inherent issues with the planned curriculum should be addressed.

Part of the 'learned curriculum' is the 'hidden curriculum'. This can be thought of as the outcomes that are not part of the explicit intentions of those planning a curriculum. These may be knowledge and skills but more importantly may be attitudes and beliefs. The formal curriculum is described in the course documents, prospectus and study guides. The hidden or unofficial curriculum is determined by the educational environment and relates to the students' experiences. There may be conflict, particularly in relation to the ethical issues between the hidden curriculum and what

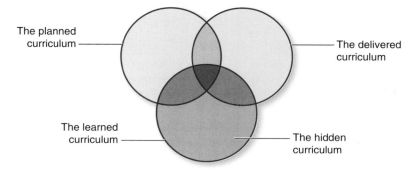

Figure 12.2 The 'planned', the 'delivered' and the 'learned' curriculum

is taught in the formal curriculum. The authentic curriculum addresses what is planned, what is taught and what is learned.

Over to you

Reflect and react

1. How familiar are you with the details of the students' curriculum in your school?
2. Would you describe your curriculum as an authentic curriculum?
3. How closely aligned are the planned and delivered curriculum?
4. How important in your context is the hidden curriculum?

Explore further

Journal articles

Bleakley, A., Bligh, J., 2008. Students learning from patients: let's get real in medical education. Adv. Health Sci. Educ. Theory Pract. 13, 89–107.

Boursicot, K., Etheridge, L., Setna, Z., et al., 2011. Performance in assessment: consensus statement and recommendations from the Ottawa conference. Med. Teach. 33, 370–383.

Brown, J.S., Collins, A., Duguid, P., 1989. Situated cognition and the culture of learning. Educ. Res. 18, 32–42.

Cooper, K., 2014. Six common mistakes that undermine motivation. Kappan 95, 11–17.

Davis, M.H., Harden, R.M., 2003. Planning and implementing an undergraduate medical curriculum: the lessons learned. Med. Teach. 25, 596–608.

Dornan, T., 2005. Osler, Flexner, apprenticeship and 'the new medical education. J. R. Soc. Med. 98, 91–95.

Rule, A.C., 2006. Editorial: The components of authentic learning. J. Auth. Learn. 3, 1–10.

Yardley, S., Brosnan, C., Richardson, J., 2013. The consequences of authentic early experience for medical students: creation of metis. Med. Educ. 47, 109–119.

Books

Grant, J., 2014. Principles of curriculum design. In: Swanwick, T. (Ed.), Understanding Medical Education: Evidence, Theory and Practice. Wiley–Blackwell, Chichester. (Chapter 3).

Hafferty, F.W., Castellani, B., 2009. The hidden curriculum: a theory of medical education. In: Brosnan, C., Turner, B.S.

(Eds.), Handbook of the Sociology of Medical Education. Routledge, London, pp. 15–35.

Kelly, A.V., 2004. The Curriculum: Theory and Practice, fifth ed. Sage, London.
A classic book on the curriculum. Although more focused on the curriculum in schools, the ideas and concepts have relevance to medical education.

Krajcik, J.S., Blumenfeld, P.C., 2006. Project based learning. In: Sawyer, R.K. (Ed.), The Cambridge Handbook of the Learning Sciences, second ed. Cambridge University Press, New York, pp. 475–488.

*Planning and implementing a curriculum requires careful atten-
tion to detail. Ten questions provide a useful checklist.*

The ten questions

Curriculum development is a serious business that requires careful consideration
and planning. In this chapter we highlight ten questions that need to be addressed:

1. What is the medical school or training programme's vision or mission?
2. What are the expected learning outcomes?
3. What content should be included?
4. How should the content be organised?
5. What educational strategies should be adopted?
6. What teaching methods should be used?
7. How should assessment be carried out?
8. How should details of the curriculum be communicated?
9. What educational environment or climate should be fostered?
10. How should the process be managed?

What is the medical school or training programme's vision or mission?

What sort of doctor does the school aim to produce? If the school was a car factory would
its programme be designed to produce economy cars, family saloons, luxury limou-
sines, sports cars or off-the-road four-wheel drives? Is it the future teacher or academic,
the research worker or the doctor who is able to work with the local community?
Perhaps all of them. In Australia, Canada, Scotland and other countries there is a need
for doctors to work in rural areas. Is there sufficient emphasis given in medical school
to prepare doctors to practise in rural communities? To what extent do students' cultural and ethnic backgrounds mirror the population they have to serve after graduation? Are medical schools responding to the challenges presented by globalisation and
international dimensions of medical practice? Schools need to recognise that there is
now a greater mobility in the medical workforce and doctors need to have the necessary
skills to function effectively in whatever part of the world they are working.

In a consideration of the vision for a medical school a question needs to be asked about the social accountability of the school. Over the last decade the concept of social accountability of medical schools has gained momentum. As defined by WHO (Boelen 1995), social accountability places 'the obligation of medical schools to direct their education, research and service activities towards addressing the priority health needs of the community, region, and/or nation they have a mandate to serve'. Social accountability is recognised in the ASPIRE-to-excellence initiative where international excellence in medical education in a school is recognised and the criteria for social accountability are specified (http://www.aspire-to-excellence.org).

Marrying a curriculum with the school's vision is often ignored or taken for granted. There is merit in taking a step back and considering how this vision impacts on the design of the curriculum in terms of the learning outcomes, the approach to teaching, learning and assessment, and the educational environment created.

What are the expected learning outcomes?

Key to a curriculum are the learning outcomes. We highlighted in Section 2 the importance of learning outcomes and the move away from an emphasis on the *education process* to an outcome-based education model where the emphasis is on *the product*. We looked at how learning outcomes can be described as they relate to technical competencies and clinical skills; approaches to practice embracing an understanding of the basic sciences, appropriate attitudes and decision-making strategies; and personal development and professionalism. Decisions about the learning outcomes should inform the answers to the questions that follow.

What content should be included?

With the rapid expansion of medical and scientific knowledge and the development of new specialties, information overload is now a major problem facing medical education. While the content has expanded significantly, the time available in the curriculum has remained relatively constant. Attempts to shoehorn more and more information into the time available with an already overloaded curriculum are self-defeating. More content can lead to less learning. Decisions need to be taken regarding what to include in the core curriculum and what to omit. There has been considerable debate, for example, about the coverage of anatomy and other basic sciences in the undergraduate curriculum and whether the level of detail could be curtailed without jeopardising the student's understanding of the subjects as related to the practice of medicine.

Decisions about what to include at each stage of training must be taken in light of the agreed learning outcomes and, as described in Chapter 12, the need for authenticity in the curriculum. There is a core content which has to be mastered by all students. Opportunities to study subjects in more depth through electives or student-selected courses should also be provided, as described in Chapter 20. Also discussed is the idea of 'threshold concepts' – difficult concepts that are essential for the student to master.

Doctors can now readily access information through the Internet and other sources when they require it. In the past the situation was very different. The emphasis was on knowing everything and believing that you knew everything. The core content curriculum must provide students with the vocabulary, understanding and skills necessary to identify and interpret information gained online and elsewhere.

How should the content be organised?

With the learning outcomes and the content determined, the next step is to consider how the curriculum should be organised and the content sequenced. The traditional approach in medical education has been to introduce students first to the basic medical sciences and normal function, structure and behaviour of the human body. As students progressed through the curriculum to the later years, the focus was on abnormal function and the development of clinical skills. Later, students developed their clinical competence on the job as they managed patients. This sequence, while having much to commend it, has major disadvantages. In the early years with a focus on the basic sciences, the relevance of the content was not obvious to the student and, as we discussed in Chapter 3, the learning may be less effective. There are alternative ways of sequencing the content that lead to more effective and efficient learning as students progress through their training. This is important and is covered in Chapter 14.

What educational strategies should be adopted?

The educational strategy adopted may be seen as the key element in a curriculum, with the curriculum even labelled in terms of the dominant educational strategy, for example a 'problem-based curriculum' or 'a community-based school'. The SPICES model for curriculum planning identifies six educational approaches and presents each on a continuum (Figure 13.1). The most appropriate point on each continuum

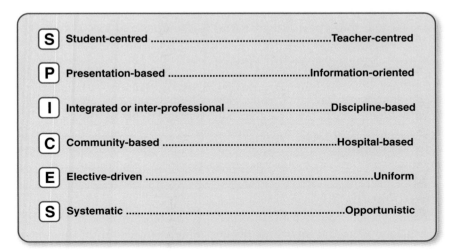

Figure 13.1 The SPICES model of educational strategies

is likely to be somewhere between the two polar points. An assessment by staff and students of the school's position on each dimension may be a useful step in planning a curriculum. The SPICES model can be used also for curriculum evaluation with the current position on the continua compared with the desired or optimum position for the school.

Student-centred/teacher-centred

There has been a significant move towards a more student-centred approach in the curriculum, as described in Chapter 15, with students given more responsibility for their own learning. It is what students learn that matters and not what teachers teach. Teachers are also being challenged and programmes scrutinised to establish whether they are meeting the needs of individual students in terms of content, approaches to learning and time taken to complete.

Presentation-based/information-orientated

A problem-based approach to learning has been adopted by a number of schools over the past two decades. The starting-off point and the focus for the learning is a clinical problem. It is what the students need to know to understand the problem that drives the activities. The curriculum can be structured around the problems with which patients present. This is discussed further in Chapter 16.

Integrated/discipline-based

There has been a significant move away from curricula based on courses that relate to individual subjects or disciplines such as anatomy, surgery and pathology, to courses integrated around the body systems, such as the cardiovascular system (Chapter 17). There is also a move towards a significantly greater integration between the basic medical sciences and clinical subjects. An interprofessional approach where different professions share, to a greater or lesser extent, their learning experiences is being explored and implemented in some education programmes. This makes sense given the need for students to develop teamwork skills. Integration and interprofessional education is explored further in Chapters 17 and 18.

Community-based/hospital-based

There has been a move away from a curriculum that provides only a hospital-based setting for students to gain their experience. More attractive is a curriculum that offers, in addition, experience in a community setting. This is covered in Chapter 19. In the past there has been a mismatch between the students' experience in the hospital setting where they receive the majority of their training and their experience in community settings where most patients receive their health care.

Elective/uniform

A curriculum should include both core elements common to all students, and electives or student-selected components. By designing a curriculum in this way there are advantages for students who can study topics of their choice, as described in Chapter 20.

Systematic (planned)/apprenticeship (opportunistic)

In a systematic approach to a curriculum there is a clear statement of the learning outcomes, and the teaching, learning and assessment is planned and related to the outcomes. This is in contrast to an opportunistic apprenticeship model where lecturers address whatever topic is of interest to them and students' experiences in a clinical attachment depend on the patients they see as they present during the attachment.

What teaching methods should be used?

After decisions have been taken about the expected learning outcomes and the educational strategies to be adopted, consideration should be given to the teaching methods used. The last decade has seen a reexamination of traditional teaching methods such as the lecture with a greater emphasis on small group work and independent learning, on the use of new learning technologies, including simulation and e-learning, and on learning in different clinical contexts. Attention has also been paid to peer-assisted learning, where students are formally involved in the education of their peers or more junior students.

The teacher's toolkit

A competent carpenter or joiner has a toolkit with a range of tools, each of which has a key function for which it has been designed. A hammer is used to insert nails. Pliers could be used for the task but they are less efficient. The toolkit will include several types of saws, each suited to their own task. With time, the carpenter will replace old tools with new improved versions that incorporate the latest technology. If we employ a carpenter, we will expect him to have a comprehensive toolkit with the appropriate tools to tackle the job for which he has been engaged. Replace 'carpenter' with 'teacher' and the situation should be no different. The teacher should have a comprehensive up-to-date range of tools for teaching and learning. Students or trainees have the right to expect that we will incorporate in our teaching the methods most appropriate for the stated learning outcomes.

In Section 4 we highlight the key tools in the teacher's toolkit, including new approaches such as the 'flipped classroom'. Much of a student's education today takes place away from the lecture theatre and the tutorial room. Today's students are very different from those of previous generations and they learn at home and informally from each other. Networking and collaborative learning play an important part in their studies.

How should assessment be carried out?

A key element in the curriculum and one that significantly influences students' behaviour is assessment. It is essential, as shown in rubrics or blueprints, that assessment matches closely the expected learning outcomes.

Decisions have to be taken about the overall assessment strategy and the appropriate instruments to be adopted with this in mind. The Objective Structured Clinical Examination (OSCE) and assessment portfolios were introduced to meet the need for more authentic and performance-based assessment instruments. Work-based assessment has grown in popularity, particularly in postgraduate education. Attention has also been paid to a closer integration of assessment and learning with the associated concept of 'assessment-for-learning' as well as 'assessment-of-learning'. Section 5 describes established and newer approaches to assessment and the key issues that have to be addressed when an assessment programme is planned. This includes setting appropriate standards.

How should details of the curriculum be communicated?

With the increased sophistication of the undergraduate and postgraduate curriculum and the use of strategies such as problem-based learning and integration, students and trainees require assistance with understanding:

- what is expected of them
- the learning opportunities available
- how they can make best use of the learning opportunities
- their progress through the curriculum.

Teachers and trainers, too, may have difficulty in grasping their role in the process and in appreciating what is expected of their students in the phase of the programme for which they have a responsibility.

If the curriculum is to succeed, teachers and students need to know what is expected of them. There is a need for a curriculum document that includes:

- a clear statement and explanation of the expected learning outcomes
- a series of blueprints relating the learning outcomes to the available learning opportunities, the phases of the curriculum and the assessment
- a curriculum map, as described in Chapter 22, that shows the relationship between the different elements in the curriculum.

What educational environment or climate should be fostered?

Important, but often ignored in the consideration of the curriculum, is the educational climate or environment. This represents the overall atmosphere students experience wherever learning takes place. It embraces, for example, the extent to which students feel they are studying in a supportive or threatening environment and whether the environment encourages teamwork and collaboration, appropriate professional behaviour, and creativity. A number of instruments are available that allow the educational environment to be measured. This topic is discussed in Chapter 21.

How should the process be managed?

It should be obvious by now that the development and management of a curriculum is an important and demanding activity that requires careful planning and allocation of time and resources. Most medical schools and postgraduate bodies have recognised this and have set up committees charged with responsibility for the curriculum. A curriculum planning committee should represent all stakeholders. Both hospital- and community-based interests should be represented and junior and senior staff and students should be included.

Individual members of staff should be allocated responsibility for implementing the different aspects of the programme including:

- the coordination of each phase in the curriculum
- the organisation and delivery of each course
- the management of electives and options
- student assessment
- support for students, including students with difficulties
- computer and information technology
- a clinical skills centre and the use of simulators and simulated patients.

It is important that staff who contribute to the education programme are recognised and rewarded for their efforts by promotion on the basis of their contribution to teaching and the scholarship of education.

Educational programmes that are most successful have strong leadership from deans or clinical directors, with support given by them for changes and innovations in the curriculum.

Over to you

Reflect and react

1. Think about the ten questions as they relate to your own teaching situation. You may not be a member of a curriculum committee or directly involved with curriculum planning, but as a stakeholder you have an important role to play and will be able to discharge your responsibilities more effectively if you have an understanding of the issues involved.
2. Think about the educational strategies for the educational programme with which you are involved. Where do you lie on the SPICES continuum and where would you like to be?

Explore further

Journal articles

Fleiszer, D.M., Posel, N.H., 2003. Development of an undergraduate medical curriculum: the McGill experience. Acad. Med. 78, 265–269.

Harden, R.M., 1986. Ten questions to ask when planning a course or curriculum. Med. Educ. 20, 356–365.

Harden, R.M., Sowden, S., Dunn, W.R., 1984. Some educational strategies in curriculum development: the SPICES model. ASME Medical Education Booklet No. 18. Med. Educ. 18, 284–297.

Stoddart, H.A., Brownfield, E.D., Churchward, G., Eley, J.W., 2016. Interweaving curriculum committees: a new structure to facilitate oversight and sustain innovation. Acad. Med. 91, 48–53.

Strasser, R., Worley, P., Cristobal, F., et al., 2015. Putting communities in the driver's seat: the realities of community-engaged medical education. Acad. Med. 90, 1466–1470.

Report

Boelen, C., 1995. Defining and Measuring the Social Accountability of Medical Schools. World Health Organisation, Geneva.

Sequencing curriculum content and the spiral curriculum 14

Sequencing curriculum content can prove complex. Some approaches to help the learner achieve the expected learning outcomes may be more effective than others.

The importance of sequencing

In planning a curriculum much attention is paid to the different elements, including the learning outcomes, the content covered, the teaching and learning methods, educational strategies and assessment. It is just as important to consider the bigger picture of the curriculum and which courses are included, and how they are sequenced. Sequencing of courses in the curriculum involves:

- *The arrangement of courses in a specific order.* The order of courses can help students to organise meaningful patterns in the vast amount of content. By doing so they are less likely to forget what they have learned and are able to apply knowledge to new problems or unfamiliar contexts. For example, the earlier introduction of clinical experiences in the curriculum provides students with a context for learning the basic sciences. The sequence of courses, however, may be dictated by the fact that prerequisites for a course may include the learning outcomes achieved in an earlier course.
- *Establishing connectivity and interdependence of the courses.* Students should be assisted in identifying connections between courses in terms of what they are currently learning, what they have previously learned and what they have still to learn. This should be made explicit in a curriculum map, as described in Chapter 22.

Guidelines for sequencing

Of prime consideration in the sequencing of courses are:

- *the prerequisites* – the knowledge or skills that the students need before entering the course
- *the course content* – what the students are required to study to master the expected learning outcomes

- *application of the competencies gained* – students' continued learning following the course

Curriculum sequencing involves managing the students' learning route in a way that makes it easier for them to achieve the learning outcomes. This may involve moving from:

- the simple to the complex
- general information or principles to a more detailed consideration
- basic principles to applications in practice

The progression from basic principles to practice, however, does not necessarily represent the optimum learning sequence for the student. If the students fail to see the relevance of courses to their ultimate goals they may lack motivation and learning may be ineffective. This is one reason for the move to introduce clinical courses and experiences earlier in the curriculum. It should also be noted that the logical ordering of content that is already obvious to a subject specialist is not necessarily the most appropriate way for a student to learn the subject.

In some situations the sequencing of courses may be influenced by logistics. For instance in clinical rotations students may undertake clinical specialty attachments in different sequences, not all being optimal.

Basic and clinical sciences

An important issue in sequencing relates to the relationship between the basic sciences and the clinical subjects. In the traditional undergraduate curriculum it was assumed that students should first acquire an understanding of the structure and function of the body before they considered pathology and clinical medicine. Students commenced their medical studies with courses relating to the basic medical sciences and, having completed these, progressed to clinically based courses. In recent years this sequence of courses in the curriculum has been questioned. Early clinical experience has been shown to have major advantages. By demonstrating relevance it motivates students and leads to more effective learning of the basic sciences. It orientates the medical curriculum towards the social context of medicine and eases students' transition to the clinical environment. It also influences students' career choice.

There is a strong argument for continuing the study of basic medical sciences into the later years of the course. Peter Garland, former professor of biochemistry at the University of Dundee, proposed that the biochemistry courses be scheduled in the later years of the curriculum rather than the early years. He believed that with this sequence students would be better equipped to appreciate the importance of the biochemistry they were studying.

A spiral curriculum

Relevant to the concept of sequencing is the idea of a spiral curriculum where there is an iterative revisiting of topics, subjects or themes (Figure 14.1). More effective

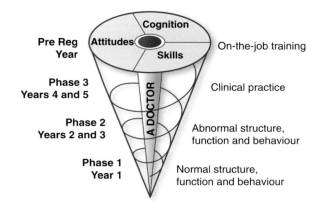

Figure 14.1   An example of a spiral curriculum
Modified *from Harden and Stamper 1999*

learning can result when the learning content is presented in smaller chunks and these are revisited later rather than when the content is presented in one larger chunk. Learning over time ('spaced learning') occurs, for example, when the cardiovascular system is considered in phase 1 of the curriculum and revisited again in phases 2 and 3. This helps to ensure that the information and understanding gained is not degraded.

A spiral curriculum is not simply the repetition of the topic taught. It requires the deepening of understanding, with each successive encounter building on the previous one. The following are the features of a spiral curriculum:

- *Topics are revisited.* Students revisit topics, themes or subjects on a number of occasions during a course. A body system such as the cardiovascular system may be studied in the early years and again at later stages in the curriculum.
- *There are increasing levels of difficulty.* The topics visited are addressed in successive levels of difficulty. Each return visit has added learning outcomes and presents fresh learning opportunities to help the student work towards the final learning outcomes.
- *New learning is related to previous learning.* New information or skills introduced are related back and linked directly to learning in previous phases of the spiral. For example, a cardiovascular system course in year 3 of a curriculum will build on the understanding of normal structure and function achieved in the cardiovascular course in year 1. In a third loop in the spiral, in the final year students have the opportunity to study cardiovascular problems in the context of patients they see in their clinical attachments.
- *Competence of students increases.* The learner's competence increases with each visit until the final learning outcomes are achieved.

Progression

The sequence of courses in the curriculum should enable students to progress effectively towards the exit learning outcomes, with the learning outcomes at each stage being challenging and achievable. This should include the development of the student's identity as a doctor.

Four dimensions can be considered in relation to students' progression through the curriculum:

- *Increased breadth.* As they progress through the programme, the learners can extend their area of competence to new topics and to different practice contexts. In clinical medicine, for example, they can learn about heart murmurs not previously considered and learn about the situation in children as distinct from adults.
- *Increased difficulty.* Students can progress by gaining a greater understanding through addressing a learning outcome in more depth. They may learn more about the pathogenesis of a disease or be able to interpret an atypical example of a cardiac murmur already studied.
- *Increased utility and application to practice.* Students can progress from a more theoretical understanding of a subject to its application in medical practice. In the early years students may practise communication skills with their colleagues or with simulated patients. In the later years they move on to communicate with patients in a range of clinical settings, at first supervised and later unsupervised.
- *Increased proficiency.* Students may demonstrate increased proficiency associated with more efficient and effective performance. This may be exemplified by less time required for a clinical task or the achievement of higher standards with fewer errors.

The four dimensions are described in Appendix 3.

Transition between courses

As students progress through the curriculum it is important that the transitions between the different phases or courses are as seamless as possible. To facilitate this, a bridging programme may be necessary. Transition or bridging courses may take into account students' individual achievements and competencies and ensure that they have the prerequisites necessary for the next step in their training programme. Should deficiencies be identified, learning opportunities can be provided to fill the gaps. Transition programmes are particularly important at the interface between undergraduate and postgraduate programmes when students take up their first medical appointment as trainee doctors. Such a programme may include a period of shadowing a junior doctor in post or a review of the practical skills expected of a junior doctor with remediation where necessary. Induction programmes can also introduce the new doctor to administrative and procedural arrangements and to other members of the team.

Over to you

Reflect and react

1. Think of your own course in the context of a spiral curriculum. Does it help students to build on what they already know? What will your course add?
2. If students fail to master the learning outcomes for your course, is there a remediation plan in place to help them before they move on to the next phase of their training?
3. Is there a need for an orientation or transitional course between your own course and what precedes or follows it?

Explore further

Journal articles

Dornan, T., Littlewood, S., Margolis, S.A., et al., 2006. How can experience in clinical and community settings contribute to early medical education? A BEME systematic review. BEME Guide No. 6. Med. Teach. 28, 13–18.

Harden, R.M., 2007. Learning outcomes as a tool to assess progression. Med. Teach. 29, 678–682.

Harden, R.M., Stamper, N., 1999. What is a spiral curriculum? Med. Teach. 21, 141–143.

Harden, R.M., Davis, M.H., Crosby, J.R., 1997. The new Dundee medical curriculum: a whole that is greater than the sum of the parts. Med. Educ. 31, 264–271.
A case study of a spiral curriculum in action.

Jarvis-Selinger, S., Pratt, D.D., Regehr, G., 2012. Competency is not enough: integrating identity formation into the medical education discourse. Acad. Med. 87, 1185–1190.
The development, over time, of a student's identity as a doctor.

Masters, K., Gibbs, T., 2007. The spiral curriculum: implications for online learning. BMC Med. Educ. 7 (52), doi:10.1186/1472-6920-7-52.
Students use of previous online resources to assist their later understanding.

The role of the teacher has to change when we empower students to take more responsibility for their own learning.

The move from teacher-centred to student-centred learning

The two key players in the medical school are the students and the teachers. There has been a significant shift in emphasis from the teacher to the student and from what is taught to what the student learns. In this move from teacher-centred to student-centred learning, the role of the teacher has changed from one of information provider to a facilitator of learning – from being a 'sage on the stage' to a 'guide on the side' (Figure 15.1). Carl Rogers, in his text *Freedom to Learn*, described 'the shift in power from the expert teacher to the student learner ... driven by a need for change in the traditional environment where students become passive, apathetic and bored'.

This concept of student-centred learning, as demonstrated in the FAIR principles described in Chapter 3, underpins much of what this book is about. A teacher-centred approach emphasises prescribed learning experiences, courses or programmes designed for the class of students with a set range of formal activities. It can be likened to eating in a restaurant with a table d'hôte menu where the diners have to eat what the restaurateur chooses. The student-centred approach in contrast is more like an à la carte menu where the diners choose what they want to eat from a menu of options provided. Teacher-centred and student-centred learning differ with regard to the student's engagement with content, the teaching and learning methods, the responsibility for learning, assessment and the balance of power (Table 15.1).

Reasons for the move

The move to student-centred learning has taken place for a number of reasons:

- Student-centred learning prepares the students to take responsibility for their continuing learning after completion of undergraduate and postgraduate studies.

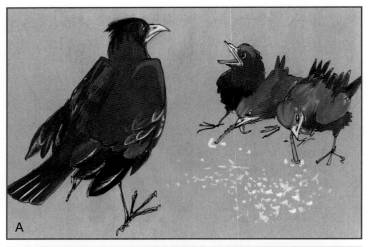

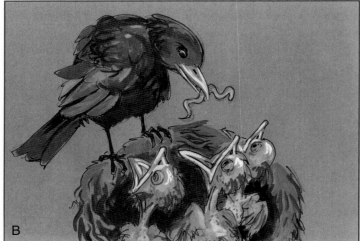

Figure 15.1 The teacher is a facilitator of learning (A) rather than an information provider (B)

- Student-centred learning is more effective and more motivating for students. As Winston Churchill said, 'Personally, I am always ready to learn, although I do not always like being taught.'
- In today's consumer-driven society there is interest in the student as both a consumer of learning and a partner in the learning process.
- Students are admitted to study medicine from more diverse backgrounds with varying learning needs.
- The concept of outcome-based education embraces a commitment to ensure that all students achieve the expected learning outcomes. What the students learn matters. How they do this will vary from student to student.
- New learning technologies, as described in Section 4, are available which give students more control over their learning.

Table 15.1 A comparison between student-centred and teacher-centred learning

	Teacher-centred	Student-centred
Underlying principle	What matters is what the teacher teaches	What matters is what the student learns
Responsibility for learning	The teacher takes responsibility for teaching and assumes the student will learn	The teacher provides the students with increasing responsibility for their own learning
Engagement with content	Students acquire content as presented by teacher	Students reflect on the content and make their own sense out of it
Relation of the teaching and learning methods to the student's achievement of the learning outcomes	The teacher does not relate the teaching to the student's achievement of the outcomes	The teacher uses a variety of methods and matches these to the student's achievement of the learning outcomes
Individualised learning	Students adapt to the curriculum	The curriculum adapts to the students
Balance of power	Decisions about the course, the approaches adopted, the policies and the deadlines are decided by the teacher	The student is engaged with decisions about the curriculum

Source: Adapted from Blumberg, P., 2009. Developing Learner-Centred Teaching: A Practical Guide for Faculty. Jossey–Bass, San Francisco

What is student-centred learning?

Student-centred learning is a system of learning that has the student at its heart. It has these elements;

- students take responsibility for their own learning
- learning is personalised to the needs of the individual students
- there is a shift in the power relationship from the teacher to the student.

Students take responsibility for their own learning

Independent learning is an important strategy in the curriculum. It is valued by students, as shown in the example in Box 15.1 when students studied endocrinology learning materials rather than attend lectures on the subject.

Student-centred learning applies aspects of self-regulation theory (Sandars and Cleary 2011). This includes:

- goal setting by the learners, which energises them and guides their actions
- monitoring and evaluating their own learning
- adjusting their learning strategy as appropriate.

> **Box 15.1** Extracts from the diary of a student studying a course where lectures were replaced with independent learning resource material
>
> **At the beginning of the course:**
>
> 'What, no lectures?'
>
> **1 week later:**
>
> 'I would prefer a lecture course with the optional extra of working on the computer.'
>
> **2 weeks later:**
>
> 'I would now choose a course combining e-learning with printed material and occasional lectures.'
>
> **4 weeks later:**
>
> 'I believe the lecture course should be scrapped. It is a waste of time. I learn better at my own rate on the computer. Now I have time to learn about endocrinology instead of just collecting a set of lecture notes.'

Student-centred learning does not mean that the teacher abandons the students to their own devices. 'Self-directed learning' (SDL) has been used to describe the approach. A more appropriate term is 'directed self-learning', as students need some form of help or guidance from the teacher, either face to face or through study guides.

Rowntree (1990) has equated a study guide to a tutor sitting on the student's shoulders, available 24 hours a day as required. The guide can be in print form or more usually is made available electronically. Its purpose is to facilitate learning by describing how the student can best interact with the range of learning opportunities available in order to meet the expected learning outcomes.

Study guides

A study guide has three elements

1. *A management function.* Students are offered advice about what they should be learning – the learning outcomes – and the range of learning opportunities available.
2. *A set of activities.* Activities embedded in the guide can require a student to apply their newly acquired knowledge and skills in practice, whether it is with a simulated patient scenario or in a real clinical context.
3. *Content.* It may contain information about the topic not readily available from another source. A study guide should not replace a textbook.

An example of a page from a study guide is given in Appendix 4.

Learning is personalised to the needs of the individual student

A development of student-centred learning is the concept of adaptive learning. In medicine a patient's management is tailored to the needs of the individual patient. Some patients with hyperthyroidism are treated with antithyroid drugs, others with radioactive iodine or surgery. Today there is a move towards more personalised medicine and in education we should follow this example by personalising or tailoring learning to match the needs of the individual student.

The delivery of personalised or adaptive learning is likely to be a significant development in the years ahead, meeting the needs of the individual student in terms of:

- what is learned – selected content in relation to learning outcomes and depth of study
- how it is learned – e.g. problem-based or directive
- when it is learned – e.g. 'just-in-time' learning
- with whom the learning occurs – collaborative learning
- where learning takes place – in class, at home or on the internet.

One of the four key recommendations of the Carnegie Foundation review of medical education in the United States was to 'provide greater options for individualizing the learning experience for students and residents' (Cooke et al. 2010).

An adaptive curriculum recognises that the student body is not a homogeneous group and that students differ in their preferred learning styles, interests and abilities. When students are provided with a range of learning opportunities and advice from the teacher or trainer, they can select those that best suit their personal needs.

It could be argued that medical schools and postgraduate training programmes are too rigid, leaving little room for students or trainees to follow their own interests and select a learning strategy that suits them. With the use of new technologies and e-learning, an almost infinite range of experiences can be provided for students to address their individual needs.

Students had choices how they learned in a blended learning cardiovascular system course in Dundee (Khogali et al. 2011). They could choose to learn individually or in pairs, to assess their understanding at the beginning or at the end of the programme and to read text or listen to an audio commentary. Students could even decide when and for how long to study and at what depth. *The New England Journal of Medicine* created a platform that, based on a clinicians' learning goals and knowledge gaps, delivered the information they needed to know.

Traditionally the time allocated for a student to complete a course or curriculum is fixed. What varies is the standard learners reach. In a truly student-centred approach with outcome-based education as described in Chapter 11, what is constant is the standard reached, with the variable being the time taken for the student to reach the standard. In this way, the course accommodates both the slow and the fast learner.

A shift of power relationship from the teacher to the student

Students should no longer be regarded simply as consumers of the education programme but as partners in the process. The term 'student engagement' refers not only to students' engagement with their studies but also to their engagement with their medical school, its curriculum, quality assurance, teaching practices and their colleagues. Students can be change agents in an institution. The 'student voice' in the medical school should be heard in:

- discussions about the mission of the medical school
- the development and implementation of the curriculum
- the evaluation of the curriculum
- the evaluation of the teachers and staff promotion
- staff development activities
- peer teaching
- its development of learning resources
- policy decisions relating, for example, to the professional behaviour of students.

Criteria for student engagement in a medical school are described in the ASPIRE-to-excellence initiative (http://www.aspire-to-exellence.org).

Over to you

Reflect and react

1. While most teachers believe that students should assume responsibility for their own learning, their behaviour as a teacher does not support this philosophy. Where does your own approach lie on the continuum between student-centred and teacher-centred approaches?
2. Think what you might be able to do in your situation to make your programme more student-centred, for example in the dimensions noted in Figure 15.1.
3. If your course lacks a study guide why not prepare one yourself? Your students will greatly appreciate your efforts.
4. The implementation in your curriculum of a fully adaptive curriculum may not yet be possible. Think, however, about the actions you might take to align the teaching and learning programme more closely to the individual needs of each student or trainee.
5. Consider the extent to which students are engaged with decisions about the curriculum and teaching programme in your school.

Explore further

Journal articles

Cullen, R., Harris, M., 2009. Assessing learner-centredness through course syllabi. Ass. Eval. High. Educ. 34, 115–125.
A description of a rubric used to assess student-centred learning in an institution.
Khogali, S.E.O., Davies, D.A., Donnan, P.T., et al., 2011. Integration of e-learning resources into a medical school curriculum. Med. Teach. 33, 311–318.
A case study of blended learning where the student has choices as to how they learn.
Murad, M.H., Coto-Yglesias, F., Varkey, P., et al., 2010. The effectiveness of self-directed learning in health professions

education: a systematic review. Med. Educ. 44, 1057–1068.

A review of the literature suggests that SDL in health professions education is associated with moderate improvement in the knowledge domain compared with traditional teaching methods.

Guides

Harden, R.M., Laidlaw, J.M., Hesketh, E.A., 1999. Study guides – their use and preparation. AMEE Medical Education Guide No. 16. Med. Teach. 21, 248–265.

Sandars, J., Cleary, T.J., 2011. Self-regulation theory: applications to medical education. AMEE Guide No. 58. Med. Teach. 33, 875–886.

Books

Blumberg, P., 2009. Developing Learner-Centred Teaching: A Practical Guide for Faculty. Jossey–Bass, San Francisco.

Cooke, M., Irby, D.M., O'Brien, B.C., 2010. Educating Physicians: A Call for Reform of Medical School and Residency. Jossey–Bass, San Francisco.

A review of medical education in the United States.

Dron, J., 2007. Control and Constraint in E-Learning, Choosing When to Choose. Idea Group Publishing, London.

A useful account of when students should be given autonomy of their learning.

Rogers, C., 1983. Freedom to Learn for the 80s. Merrill, Ohio.

A classic text on student-centred learning.

Rowntree, D., 1990. Teaching Through Self-Instruction. Kogan Page Ltd, London.

Websites

ASPIRE. 2015. ASPIRE Recognition of Excellence in Student Engagement in a Medical, Dental and Veterinary School: An Introduction. http://www.aspire-to-excellence.org/downloads/1123/ASPIRE.

An account of student engagement and how this is assessed in the ASPIRE-to-excellence programme.

Christensen, U.J., 2015. Adaptive learning and medical education. https://www.aacc.org/~/media/transcripts/clinical-chemistry-journal/podcasts/2015/adaptive-learning-and-medical-education.pdf.

Smart technology that adapts to clinicians' learning goals and knowledge gaps to deliver the information they need to know.

Gibbs, G., 2014. Student engagement, the latest buzzword. https://www.timeshighereducation.co.uk/news/student-engagement-the-latest-buzzword/2012947.article.

An examination of what is implied with the use of the term 'student engagement'.

A clinical problem or task undertaken by a healthcare professional can serve as the basis for learning. The student is motivated by the more authentic learning experience.

The importance of the clinical problem in student learning

In the traditional curriculum, learners start with a consideration of basic and clinical sciences, then move on to the application of the theory to practice. They first learn, for example, about thyroid physiology and the hormones secreted by the gland and about the pathology of abnormalities associated with the thyroid gland. They then move on to see patients who present with a goitre or with the symptoms of underactivity or overactivity of the gland. In contrast with an integrated and problem-based approach, students start by considering patients with a thyroid problem. They have then to work out what knowledge and skills they require to assess and manage the problem.

Clinical problems can be used not only as the starting point for the students' learning in one topic but also, as in problem-based learning (PBL), a framework for the learning. In Dundee Medical School the curriculum from year 1 to 5 was structured around 104 clinical presenting problems, such as abdominal pain.

Structuring learning using clinical scenarios as a framework offers a number of advantages.

- It motivates students to understand the relevance to clinical practice of what they are learning. Relevance is part of the FAIR model, as described in Chapter 3.
- It introduces the student to clinical practice and helps to establish their personal identity as a doctor.
- It provides a basis or framework for lifelong learning.
- It facilitates future knowledge retrieval as the situation where the knowledge is learned more closely resembles the context where it is later applied.

Problem-based learning (PBL)

What is PBL?

Problem-based learning has been adopted worldwide as an education strategy in medical education. Its use, however, has not been without controversy. The principal idea behind PBL, as described above, is that the starting point for the learning is a clinical problem. This is the focus for the student's learning and drives the learning activities on a 'need to know' basis. PBL has made a major contribution to medical education, but there has been a lack of clarity or a conceptual fog surrounding what is meant by the term and how it is implemented in practice. The underpinning educational principles are:

- Students are presented with examples from clinical practice, and then work out the principles or rules from the basic and clinical sciences that allow them to understand and interpret the problem.
- Students engage actively with learning, collaborating with their colleagues in a small group. (Activity is included in the FAIR model.)
- Students learn by self-study thus ensuring they understand the subject matter. (The Individual element in the FAIR model.)

For PBL to succeed, it is essential that both students and faculty are motivated, have an understanding of these principles and accept their roles and responsibilities (Bate et al. 2014).

In PBL, approaches have varied regarding the steps in the process, the nature and format of 'the problem' and the level of support given to students. PBL is based usually on small group work, with 8–10 students per group, although larger numbers of students can be engaged. A member of staff usually facilitates the group, but students can act as facilitators. Although small group work is seen by some as an essential feature of PBL, the technique can be used in the lecture situation or with individual students working independently online.

PBL can be implemented in practice in a variety of ways. Here is one example. The sequence is normally completed over the course of a week.

1. At the first meeting of the group:
   - Students receive the problem scenario. Traditionally this has been in print format, typically a short description of a patient's presentation. The problem may be presented, however, using a multimedia approach with a computer, video tape or simulator. Simulated patients have also been used.
   - Students identify and clarify unfamiliar terms, then define and agree the issues to be discussed. It is important that students do not spend too much time figuring out what they should learn at the expense of time spent learning.
   - Students consider possible explanations of the situation presented on the basis of their prior knowledge and identify areas where further learning is

required. The tutor helps to ensure that the learning outcomes identified by the students are appropriate and match the learning outcomes for the course, and are achievable in the time available.

2. Students then work independently and gather information relating to the learning outcomes. The group may agree to subdivide the task and allocate different responsibilities to individual members. Some of this work may be done in the small group setting online using a search engine such as Google.
3. The group reconvenes and shares the results of their private study. What they learn is then applied to the problem presented.
4. Additional information about the patient may be presented to the students and the above process is repeated.

The PBL continuum

Various points have been defined on the continuum, between a problem-based approach and an information-oriented approach as described in the SPICES model (Harden and Davis 1999). This is summarised in Appendix 5.

The context for PBL

PBL is usually adopted in the context of an integrated medical curriculum but the strategy can also be used in a curriculum where the emphasis is on subjects or disciplines.

Most commonly PBL has been used in the context of the early years of undergraduate education. The strategy has a role to play also in the later years of undergraduate education and in postgraduate and continuing education, although a task-based approach, as described later in this chapter, may be more appropriate in these settings. In continuing education the doctor may work individually at a distance with problems presented online or paper-based.

PBL can also be used alongside team-based learning (TBL), as noted in Chapter 24.

Task-based learning (TkBL)

What is task-based learning?

Task-based learning has been described by Phil Race as 'a very useful approach to integration of the medical curriculum and, not least, a time-efficient and cost-effective approach to developing highly relevant skills, attributes and competences for the profession' (Race 2000).

Task-based learning (TkBL) incorporates the same educational philosophy as PBL and indeed has been described as part of the PBL continuum. In task-based learning the focus for the learner is not a paper problem simulation but the description of a task addressed by healthcare professionals. An example is 'a patient with abdominal pain' or 'a patient with breathlessness'. In task-based learning the objective is not only to learn to manage a patient with the problem but to gain a more in-depth

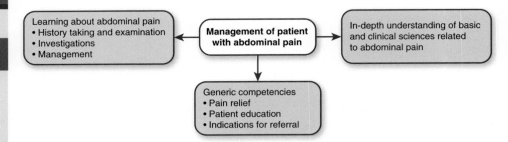

Figure 16.1 In task-based learning (TBL), learning occurs around a task

understanding of the task or problem by learning the basic and clinical sciences relevant to the problem (Figure 16.1). In the abdominal pain example, in the early years the student's attention is focused on issues such as the relevant anatomy and physiology of the abdomen, on the understanding of the mechanism of pain and on abdominal pathologies, and in the later years on the different approaches to investigation and management of a patient with abdominal pain.

TkBL in a clinical setting

TkBL is useful as an approach to deliver curriculum integration and PBL in the context of the clinical clerkships (Harden et al. 2000). In the example of 'abdominal pain', students concentrate on different aspects of the task in each of their clerkships and a wide range of learning outcomes or competencies can be addressed, such as:

- Acute abdominal pain and the emergency diagnosis and management in a surgical clerkship.
- Approaches to the investigation of a patient in a medical clerkship.
- Specific aspects relating to gynaecological causes in a gynaecological clerkship.
- Age-related differences in a geriatric or paediatric attachment.
- Psychosomatic aspects in a psychiatry attachment.
- The roles of different members of the healthcare team, early diagnosis, decision making and coping with uncertainty in a General Practice attachment. When, for example, should a patient complaining of abdominal pain be investigated and referred to hospital?
- Geographical and cultural differences in an overseas elective.

TkBL places more responsibility on the student and serves to integrate learning across a range of clinical rotations in an undergraduate curriculum or postgraduate training programme.

Implementation of TkBL

Medical schools that adopt a TkBL approach generate usually about 100 to 150 clinical presentations as the focus or framework for the curriculum. The student's understanding of the task becomes more sophisticated as he or she progresses through the curriculum. A list of the 104 presentations adopted in Dundee Medical School is given in Appendix 6.

Rubrics or blueprints should be produced that identify how each task contributes to the learning outcomes and to the range of learning experiences in which the students engage. As described above, each clinical clerkship can contribute in a different way to the student's mastery of the learning outcomes of the course.

TkBL provides a structure and focus for postgraduate education that previously was all too often lacking. It helps resolve what may be perceived to be a conflict between service delivery and the education of the student or trainee. Six tasks performed routinely by trainee dentists were identified as the basis for a postgraduate dental training programme. The expected learning outcomes were specified for each task, as illustrated in the grid in Appendix 7.

The tasks specified in the curriculum documents also provide a framework for a student's portfolio and can be used to assess their progress, as described in Chapter 33.

Clinical presentations

A similar approach to task-based learning is the 'clinical presentation' curriculum introduced in Calgary, Canada, which is based on the problems patients present to doctors (Mandin et al. 1995).

Clinical presentations were defined that represented a common or important way in which a patient, group of patients, community or population actually presents to the physician and which a graduate would be expected to deal with. The presentation identified also has to be important and substantive enough to cover a broad content so that the learning outcomes can be met. Less substantive clinical presentations were included under a broader category. For example, 'epistaxis' was included under bleeding tendency/bruising.

Both a clinical presentation curriculum and task-based learning offer students the benefit of an organisational scheme that serves as a scaffold to which they can add new information and which relates theory to practice.

A curriculum cube

As discussed in Chapter 12, a curriculum is much more than a collection of topics to be studied or a syllabus to be followed. Wragg (1997) described in *The Cubic Curriculum* three curriculum dimensions – the subject matter, cross-curricular themes and issues, and the different methods of teaching and learning. In medical education (Figure 16.2) this translates into the three dimensions of:

- the learning outcomes or competencies
- the clinical presentations and tasks
- the courses and the learning opportunities, e.g. a lecture or PBL session

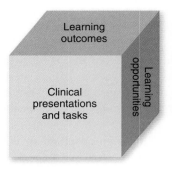

Figure 16.2 The curriculum cube. The clinical presentations and tasks are related to the learning outcomes and the learning opportunities

Each clinical presentation or task is related in the curriculum cube to the relevant learning outcomes and learning opportunities. Each learning outcome is related to the clinical presentations that contribute to the mastery of the learning outcome, and the courses and learning opportunities where it is addressed.

Over to you

Reflect and react

1. Where are you on the PBL continuum as described in Appendix 5? PBL has proved attractive as an educational strategy for many teachers who have been intent on improving their courses. Others have been reluctant to adopt a teaching approach that seems alien to what they believe to be 'good teaching'. Where do you stand?
2. If you have adopted PBL in your teaching do you make full use of the new technologies when presenting a problem to the learner?
3. Consider using a set of tasks or clinical presentations as a framework for your curriculum and relate them to the expected learning outcomes.

Explore further

Journal articles

Colliver, J.A., 2000. Effectiveness of problem-based learning curricula: research and theory. Acad. Med. 75, 259–266.

Dolmans, D., Michaelsen, L., Van Merrienboer, J., et al., 2015. Should we choose between problem-based learning and team-based learning? No, combine the best of both worlds! Med. Teach. 37, 354–359.

Harden, R.M., Davis, M.H., 1999. The continuum of problem-based learning. Med. Teach. 20, 317–322.

A model for analysing the level at which PBL is introduced into a curriculum.

Harden, R.M., Crosby, J.R., Davis, M.H., et al., 2000. Task-based learning: the answer to integration and problem-based learning in the clinical years. Med. Educ. 34, 391–397.

Mandin, H., Harasym, P., Eagle, C., et al., 1995. Developing a 'clinical presentation' curriculum at the University of Calgary. Acad. Med. 70, 186–193.

Race, P., 2000. Task-based learning. Med. Educ. 34 (5), 335–336.

A commentary on the concept of task-based learning.

Guides

Bate, E., Hommes, J., Duvivier, R., et al., 2014. Problem-based learning (PBL). Getting the most out of your students – their roles and responsibilities. AMEE Guide No. 84. Med. Teach. 36, 1–12.

Davis, M.H., Harden, R.M., 1999. Problem-Based Learning: A Practical Guide. AMEE Medical Education Guide No. 15. AMEE, Dundee.

Harden, R.M., Laidlaw, J.M., Ker, J.S., et al. 1998. Task-Based Learning: An Educational Strategy for Undergraduate, Postgraduate and Continuing Medical Education. AMEE Medical Education Guide No. 7. AMEE, Dundee.

Taylor, D., Miflin, B., 2010. Problem-Based Learning: Where Are We Now? AMEE Medical Education Guide No. 36. AMEE, Dundee.

Book

Wragg, E.C., 1997. The Cubic Curriculum. Routledge, London.

Using an integrated approach 17

An integrated curriculum bringing together different disciplines offers major advantages.

A move to an integrated curriculum

The most significant change that has taken place globally in medical education since the 1970s has been the move from curricula that focused on individual subjects or disciplines to a programme where the teaching and learning is integrated. In a traditional discipline-based curriculum, subjects were taught in separate courses, each with its own programme of lectures and its own assessment. Students learned about the structure of the heart in the anatomy course, the cardiac drugs in the pharmacology course and the abnormalities of the heart in the pathology course (Figure 17.1).

The disadvantages were highlighted by Poynter (1970):

> 'To take an industrial analogy, it is rather as if a great variety of machine tools were assembled from a number of different car factories and linked together in the belief that the ultimate product would be a motor car of some kind, although nobody was at all sure what it would look like or how it would perform.'

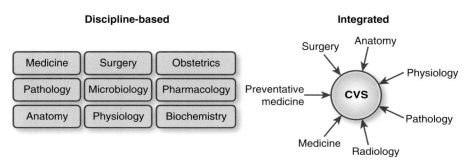

Figure 17.1 A comparison between how subjects are covered in a discipline-based and integrated curriculum relating to the cardiovascular system (CVS)

A strong departmental structure in a medical school has made integration of the curriculum more difficult. The need for integration, however, has now been widely accepted by medical schools and accrediting bodies. In the Carnegie Foundation Review of Medical Education in the United States, the importance of integration in the curriculum was featured (Cooke et al. 2010). With an integrated approach the different subjects are brought together, most typically around a body system such as the cardiovascular system. Integration has been described as the deliberate unification of separate areas of knowledge (Goldman and Schroth 2012). The term 'horizontal integration' is used to describe the bringing together of subjects in the same phase of the curriculum. 'Vertical integration' is applied to the integration of subjects normally taught in different phases of the curriculum. Traditionally, the early years of the medical course were devoted to the study of the basic medical sciences. More recently we have seen, as described in Chapter 12, the introduction of clinical learning opportunities into the earlier years with the basic sciences related to them. More attention does need to be paid to the integration of the basic sciences with clinical medicine in the later years of the curriculum.

Advantages of integration

Having emerged from the shadows as an alternative approach to curriculum development, integration has become the standard approach in many medical schools worldwide and is required by accrediting bodies. There are a number of reasons for this:

- **Integrated teaching reflects the practice of medicine**. An integrated approach, more than a discipline-based approach, encourages the student to take a holistic view of the patient and his or her problems. In a final examination in a medical school that had a discipline-based curriculum we observed that a student, when asked to take a history from a woman with abdominal pain, enquired whether he should take a medical, surgical or gynaecological history. He had clearly failed to integrate what he had learned in the different clinical attachments.
- **Integration motivates the students**. Most students are not interested in becoming anatomists or physiologists and the relevance of the basic sciences to the practice of medicine may not be appreciated by them. The traditional curriculum, sadly, was often associated in the early years with a decrease in the students' enthusiasm and interest in medicine.
- **Integration by relating theory to practice makes learning more effective**. In a classic experiment, divers learned from a text underwater and on the surface. When tested subsequently on the surface they performed better on the text learned on the surface. When tested underwater they performed better on the text they had learned underwater. This has been replicated in many other studies. The ability to retrieve an item from memory depends on the similarity between the condition in which it was learned and the context in which it is to be retrieved and applied. What matters is how students can use their basic science knowledge when managing patients rather than in a

classroom examination. It is also recognised that knowledge learned in isolation and not applied is easily forgotten – so called 'inert' knowledge.

- **An integrated curriculum can help to avoid unnecessary reduplication**. An integrated curriculum highlights what is important for the student to know and can be seen as a response to the problem of information overload.
- **The integrated curriculum may be more cost effective**. Greater efficiency can be achieved by sharing teaching and learning resources, such as the facilities in a clinical skills laboratory.
- **An integrated approach promotes collaboration and communication between staff**. Staff need to discuss how each subject can contribute to the learning outcomes. Staff who collaborate in their teaching may go on to collaborate in their research activities.

Focus for integration

An integrated curriculum may have one or more themes:

- **The body systems**. This is the most commonly adopted approach in the early years of the medical course. Students study, for example, a 6-week course on the cardiovascular system, a 5-week course on the respiratory system, etc.
- **The life cycle**. A focus for the integration may be the life cycle, including the newborn, the child, the adolescent, the adult, the elderly and the dying. This may be used in conjunction with a system-based approach.
- **Clinical presentations or a set of descriptions of the tasks facing a doctor**. Task-based learning as described in Chapter 16 and in Appendix 3 is a useful approach to integration, particularly in the later years of the course (Harden et al. 2000).

The integration continuum

Discussions about integration have been polarised, with some teachers arguing in favour and others against integrated teaching. In the SPICES model for educational strategies, integration is presented as a continuum with full integration at one end and discipline-based teaching at the other (Harden 2000). A position between the two extremes may be adopted as described on the integration ladder (Figure 17.2). This has been found to be a useful tool to explore integration in a curriculum and to identify the most appropriate level to suit a particular curriculum.

Step 1 – Isolation

Departments or subject specialists, represented by squares, organise their teaching in isolation with no consideration of other subjects or disciplines.

Step 2 – Awareness

The teaching is subject-based, as in Step 1, but some mechanisms are in place whereby a teacher in one subject is made aware of what is covered in other subjects in the curriculum.

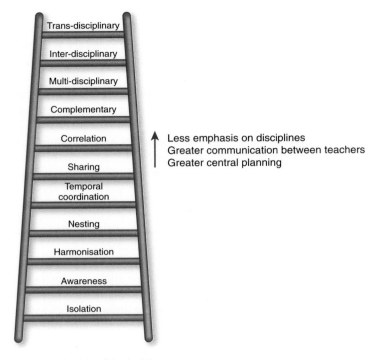

Figure 17.2 The integration ladder.
(Modified from Harden, R.M., 2000. The integration ladder: a tool for curriculum planning and evaluation. Med. Educ. 34, 551–557.)

Step 3 – Harmonisation

In harmonisation, teachers responsible for different courses consult with each other and communicate about their course.

Step 4 – Nesting

In this integrated approach the teacher includes, within a subject-based course, knowledge and skills relating to other subjects.

Step 5 – Temporal coordination

The timetable is adjusted so that related topics within subjects are scheduled at the same time, with similar topics being taught on the same day or week.

Step 6 – Sharing

Some teaching is shared between two departments or disciplines implementing the teaching programme.

Step 7 – Correlation

In addition to the subject-based teaching, an integrated teaching session is introduced that brings together areas of common interest in each of the subjects.

Step 8 – Complementary

There is both subject-based and integrated teaching but with integrated sessions representing a major feature of the curriculum.

Step 9 – Multi-disciplinary

A number of subjects are brought together in a single course with an integrated theme, but with the subjects clearly identified.

Step 10 – Inter-disciplinary

Subjects lose their identity in a new integrated programme.

Step 11 – Trans-disciplinary

The integration is built around the field of knowledge as exemplified in the real world rather than a theme or topic selected for the purpose.

Over to you

Reflect and react

1. Think about the approach to integration in your course. What is the focus for the integration and where are you on the integration ladder? You should not remain on the bottom rung of the ladder.
2. If you have an integrated curriculum, do the learning outcomes, the learning opportunities provided and the assessment all reflect an integrated approach?

Explore further

Journal articles

Goldman, E., Schroth, W.S., 2012. Deconstructing integration: a framework for the rational application of integration as a guiding curricular strategy. Acad. Med. 87, 729–734.

Harden, R.M., Crosby, J., Davis, M.H., et al., 2000. Task-based learning: the answer to integration and problem-based learning in the clinical years. Med. Educ. 34, 391–397.

Harden, R.M., 2000. The integration ladder: a tool for curriculum planning and evaluation. Med. Educ. 34, 551–557.

De Jong, P.G.M., 2015. Introduction to the theme for 2015: integration. Med. Sci. Educ. 25, 341.

An introduction to a series of papers on integration.

Books

Bandaranayake, R., 2011. The Integrated Medical Curriculum. Radcliffe Publishing, London.

Cooke, M., Irby, D.M., O'Brien, B.C., 2010. Educating Physicians. Jossey–Bass, San Francisco.

Further attention needs to be paid to integration in the curriculum.

Fogarty, R., 1991. How to Integrate the Curricula. IRI/Skylight Training and Publishing, Illinois.

Mennin, S., 2016. Integration of the sciences basic to medicine and the whole of the curriculum. In: Abdulrahman, K.A.B., Mennin, S., Harden, R.M., et al. (Eds.), Routledge International Handbook of Medical Education. Routledge, London. (Chapter 13).

Poynter, F.N.L., 1970. Medical education in England since 1600. In: O'Malley, C.D. (Ed.), The History of Medical Education. University of California Press, Los Angeles.

Interprofessional education (IPE) 18

Interprofessional education if adopted can contribute to better delivery of health care.

A move to IPE

Integrated teaching as described in Chapter 17 is concerned with bringing together the disciplines within medicine. Interprofessional education (IPE) occurs when two or more different professions learn with, from and about each other. Although its implementation is not easy, IPE now features to some extent in many curricula and is mandated or recommended by a number of accrediting bodies. There are good reasons for this (Harden 2015). If we expect a doctor on qualification to practise effectively as a member of a team and to have the required team and communication skills and an understanding and respect for other healthcare professionals, we need to reflect this in the curriculum and the educational strategies adopted.

In medical practice today, no one profession can respond adequately to the range of problems presented by patients. It is essential that doctors have the necessary team-work skills and understanding of different roles if they are to work alongside nurses, pharmacists, physiotherapists, health visitors and other members of the healthcare team. The education of doctors has been largely conducted in a silo with little consideration given to the other professions and almost no collaboration with regard to joint educational programmes. IPE enables the knowledge and skills necessary for collaborative working to be learned and can result in an improvement in the delivery of health care.

The adoption of IPE has been encouraged by the move to outcome-based education as described in Section 2 of this book and the need for a more authentic curriculum as described in Chapter 12. IPE is now being adopted across the continuum of education from the early years of the medical school, through postgraduate training to continuing professional development.

Principles of interprofessional learning

The Centre for the Advancement of Interprofessional Education (CAIPE) in the UK developed seven principles to guide the provision, commissioning and development of interprofessional education (Freeth 2014). The vision is that interprofessional education:

- works to improve the quality of care
- focuses on the needs of service users and carers
- involves service users and carers
- encourages professions to learn with, from and about each other
- respects the integrity and contribution of each profession
- enhances practice within the professions
- increases professional satisfaction.

Continuum of interprofessional education

Interprofessional education can be described along a continuum of 11 stages, from isolation, where healthcare professionals are taught separately from each other with no contact, to transprofessional education, where learning is based in practice (Harden 1998). The steps are similar to the steps described in the integration ladder in Chapter 17. A decision should be taken on where the school wishes to be on the IPE ladder. This should be higher than the first two rungs and there should be some recognition of other professions in the curriculum. With time the school may progress up the ladder.

Implementation in practice

Implementation of IPE is not easy and there are problems with regard to the timetable, location and issues relating to the curriculum. With imagination, consideration and collaboration these can usually be overcome. The possibility of success or failure can be captured with the equation noted in Chapter 6 in relation to collaboration, and applied to the context of IPE (Harden 2015).

$$IPE = (vision \times the\ implementation\ strategy)/ negative\ perceptions\ of\ the\ approach$$

Success is more likely where there is a well-thought-out and shared vision for what is to be achieved, an appropriate implementation strategy and a plan to counteract a negative mindset.

A vision for IPE

For IPE to be successful we require a clear agreed vision with achievable goals. Interprofessional education should have a vision that is imaginable, flexible, feasible, desirable, focused and communicable. Course organisers, teachers in the different professions and students need to have a common sense of purpose and a clear understanding of the rationale for the IPE and in their context what constitutes IPE.

An implementation strategy

Methods used to implement interprofessional education in practice, as described by Barr (2009), include:

- **Action-based learning**. For example, problem-based learning (PBL) and task-based learning (TkBL)
- **Exchange-based learning**. For example, debates, case studies, shared lectures and e-learning
- **Observation-based learning**. For example, joint visits to a patient by students from different professions, shadowing another profession and work-related practice placements
- **Simulation-based learning**. For example, role-play, games, skills laboratory and a simulated ward
- The use of **portfolios for learning and assessment**

Resource materials may be developed that incorporate interprofessional practice. We worked with a multiprofessional team from Africa to develop a training handbook for use by members of the healthcare team. The handbook was based on the common clinical problems encountered by healthcare professionals in their daily work, e.g. a patient with diarrhoea. A general account of the management of the problem was provided in the top half of each page. In three columns on the lower half of the page there were descriptions of the roles of the doctor, the nurse and the health officer. The team members mastered the skills relating to their own roles, while gaining an understanding of the roles of other members of the healthcare team.

How interprofessional education is implemented is important and may determine the success of the approach. In PBL multiprofessional groups may succeed or fail depending on the nature of the presenting problem, the briefing of the group, the facilitation by the tutor and the debriefing. PBL worked effectively in our experience with a group of trainee midwives and medical students when the task facing the group required both the practical experience of the trainee midwives and the theoretical understanding of the medical students. The result was a positive shift in attitude of medical students towards midwives and vice versa. Other reported experiences of multiprofessional groups where the task was less well defined and did not require the experience of the different professions have been less successful. In implementing IPE there needs to be a clear statement of the expected learning outcomes for the curriculum and how the IPE contributes to achievement of the learning outcomes.

Tackling a negative mindset

Any negative mindset of both staff and students must be tackled. The potential barriers to IPE need to be addressed at a leadership level. Views that must be rebutted and which contribute to an image problem for IPE include academic elitism, that IPE destroys individual characteristics, that there is a potential loss of professional identity, that personality conflicts are common, that IPE is not considered worth the effort and that the logistics are too difficult.

Over to you

Reflect and react

1. In the planning and implementation of your training programme, has an interprofessional approach been considered? Have you discussed this with teachers in other professions?
2. Where does your programme sit on the interprofessional ladder and where would you like it to sit?

Explore further

Journal articles

Harden, R.M., 1998. Effective multiprofessional education: a three-dimensional perspective. Med. Teach. 20, 402–408.
A description of the IPE ladder.
Harden, R.M., 2015. Interprofessional education: the magical mystery tour now less of a mystery. Anat. Sci. Educ. 8, 291–295.
Mires, G.J., Williams, F.L.R., Harden, R.M., et al., 1999. Multiprofessional education in undergraduate curricula can work. Med. Teach. 21, 281–285.
A case study of successful IPE.
Norgaard, B., Draborg, E., Vestergaard, E., et al., 2013. Interprofessional clinical training improves self-efficacy of health care students. Med. Teach. 35, e1235–e1242.
Interprofessional training improved students' perception of self-efficacy more than traditional clinical training.
Thistlethwaite, J.E., Forman, D., Matthews, L.R., et al., 2014. Competencies and frameworks in interprofessional education: a comparative analysis. Acad. Med. 86, 869–875.
There is a need to emphasise outcomes that might be attained only through interprofessional activity.

Guides

Hammick, M., Freeth, D., Koppel, I., et al., 2007. The best evidence systematic review of interprofessional education. BEME Guide No. 9. Med. Teach. 29, 735–751.
Hean, S., Craddock, D., Hammick, M., 2012. Theoretical insights into interprofessional education. AMEE Guide No. 62. Med. Teach. 34, e78–e101.

Books

Barr, H., 2009. Interprofessional education as an emerging concept. In: Bluteau, P., Jackson, A. (Eds.), Interprofessional Education: Making It Happen. Palgrave Macmillan, Basingstoke.
Forman, D., VanLeit, B., 2016. Implementing interprofessional education. In: Abdulrahman, K.A.B., Mennin, S., Harden, R.M., et al. (Eds.), Routledge International Handbook of Medical Education. Routledge, New York. (Chapter 14).
Lessons learned about IPE from case studies around the world.
Freeth, D., 2014. Interprofessional education. In: Swanwick, T. (Ed.), Understanding Medical Education: Evidence, Theory and Practice, second ed. Wiley–Blackwell, Chichester. (Chapter 6).
Thistlethwaite, J.E., 2013. Interprofessional education. In: Dent, J.A., Harden, R.M. (Eds.), A Practical Guide for Medical Teachers, fourth ed. Elsevier, London. (Chapter 23).

SECTION 3

The apprenticeship, community-based education, longitudinal clinical clerkships and work-based learning

19

There is no better way to learn than from work-related experience. This requires careful monitoring and supervision.

The apprenticeship model

In the 19th century and earlier, doctors were trained as apprentices to practising doctors. The master accepted the pupil, who paid for the privilege and was taught and instructed in the methods and secrets (Calman 2006). In the late 19th and early part of the 20th century the lack of attention to the scientific basis of medicine in undergraduate education, the lack of a formal curriculum and the varying quality of the apprenticeship experience offered led to a significant shift towards university-based education. The emphasis was placed on more formal and theoretical education in the classroom and on the didactic lecture.

Over the years there has been growing disquiet about the removal of much of the education from the clinical setting, and today greater emphasis is again being placed on learning on the job in the workplace setting, including the community. The learning experience, however, is being more carefully arranged and monitored, with on-the-job learning incorporated as part of a more formal planned curriculum.

Trends in curriculum planning

In planning a curriculum there has been a move as described in earlier chapters:

- from theory to practice and on-the-job learning with the concept of the authentic curriculum
- from hospital-based to community-based learning
- from short discipline-based attachments to longer, more integrated attachments delivered through what is described as longitudinal clinical clerkships.

In this chapter we look at community-based education, the longitudinal clinical clerkship and more generally at the concept of work-based learning.

Community-based education

What is community-based education?

In the past, medical education was almost exclusively based in a teaching hospital. The vast majority of health care, however, occurs in the community and a recurring theme in curriculum planning has been the need to move medical education from the hospital end of the SPICES continuum in the direction of the community end (see Chapter 13). Community-based education refers to medical education that is based outside a tertiary or large secondary level hospital. It is usually based in general practice but may include other community experiences or work with other healthcare providers.

Community-oriented education refers to an education programme that is designed to teach about health care in the community, with some components in the community and others in a teaching hospital.

Rationale for community-based education

Some accrediting bodies now require a curriculum to include a community-based element. There are strong reasons for including a significant emphasis in the curriculum on student experience in the community. These reasons are:

- Community-based education provides students with experience of common diseases and conditions which they may not see in the hospital context.
- Students see patients from a holistic perspective in their social context.
- Some learning outcomes are more easily achieved through a community attachment, including teamwork skills, professionalism, cultural competence and an understanding of community health problems.
- Students gain an understanding of the interactive roles that social conditions such as education, housing and economic factors have on health.
- Some students are motivated by their experience to take up their career in general practice and are helped to prepare for this.
- The involvement of the local community in the education programme for students is consistent with a social contract between the school and the local community which it serves.
- Community-based experience if integrated in the early years can be used to demonstrate the relevance of basic sciences to medical practice (Dornan et al. 2006).
- Students are facilitated in forming their identity as a doctor.
- Clinical training slots are provided in addition to those in the hospital setting which helps to accommodate the increase in the number of students admitted to study medicine.

Urban and rural settings

Community-based experiences may be offered in urban or rural settings. In Australia some medical schools have rural clinical schools where students receive a large part of their clinical training. Students learning in a rural setting have been found to perform as well as or better in examinations than students engaged with a hospital-based experience.

Implementation of community-based learning

While many medical schools now include elements of community-based education in their curriculum, a few schools have community-based education as a major curriculum focus. Schools with a commitment to community-based education are members of the *Network Towards Unity for Health.*

In implementing a community-based programme, consideration should be given to:

- A clear specification of the learning outcomes expected in relation to community-based learning. Where students have both hospital- and community-based learning there should be an indication of the learning outcomes that can be achieved more readily in the community- than the hospital-based context.
- Alignment of the assessment with the community-based experience irrespective of whether the assessment is a written examination, an OSCE or a portfolio.
- Involvement of all stakeholders including the curriculum managers and designers, the teachers in the community, patients and the local community.
- Briefing and training where necessary of teachers in the community with regard to the curriculum, the expected outcomes from the community attachment and the educational strategies adopted.
- Ensuring that Internet connections are easily available, and there is access to online learning resources by students at a distance from the medical school.
- Provision of a study guide for students to assist them in making the greatest benefit from the opportunities available.
- Making available a mentor or support for the students should this be required.
- Recognising and rewarding contributions made by local teachers to community-based teaching.

Longitudinal integrated clerkships (LICs)

The problem with the traditional clinical clerkships

The clerkship has been a major element in medical education programmes. Problems associated with the traditional hospital-based clerkship model are:

- Students see patients only for the short period of time they are in hospital and do not see the continuity of care.
- Patients, often admitted through accident and emergency departments, do not represent the wide range of minor or chronic illness.
- Access by students to patients is difficult because of the short duration of their stay in hospital or the intensity of their investigations.

- Clerkships are in different specialties with the emphasis on specialisation rather than on integrated care.
- It is difficult for students, because of the short duration of clerkships, to have a meaningful role in the delivery of patient care.

Features of a LIC

As a result of the above difficulties, LICs have been introduced to replace or complement the traditional clinical clerkship (Norris et al. 2009, Hudson et al 2016). The features of the LIC are:

- Students have a continuing relationship with patients for an extended period of time, up to one year. This highlights the importance of continuity of care.
- Students have a continuing relationship with their teachers and are able to build long-term learning relationships.
- Students participate in integrated clinical care involving a number of disciplines, professions and other members of the healthcare team.
- Students actively participate as members of the healthcare team with their learning interwoven through the continuities of patient contact and care.

Implementation of LICs

LICs are based most commonly in the community, both in urban and rural settings, but may also be based in the hospital setting and ambulatory care. In the implementation of a LIC similar issues should be addressed to those described for community-based education. The students' schedule should provide the required mix of patients and learning opportunities and should relate to the core curriculum for the school. More formal case conferences and other learning opportunities may be included. Students can engage in shared learning opportunities online with other students at different sites.

Many schools around the world have adopted LICs as an elective or option in their curriculum and some run mandatory LICs.

A *Consortium of Longitudinal Integrated Clerkships (CLIC)* provides a link with schools who have adopted or are considering adopting LICs in their curriculum.

Work-based learning

What is work-based learning?

Work-based learning (WBL) is a key strategy in postgraduate and continuing education but it is relevant too in undergraduate education. It can be seen as a continuum that stretches from formalised training at one end where a student or junior doctor learns under supervision through to an established practitioner sharing a clinical problem with colleagues as part of their continuing professional development.

A number of terms have been used to describe WBL. These include on-the-job learning (OJL), service-based learning, experience-based learning, learning from practice and situated learning. Community-based learning is often interpreted as work-based learning. The key feature is that students and trainees participate in authentic activities that form the basis for their learning. They learn from their experience and are helped to generalise from the patient they have seen to other patients and situations. Students or trainees learn 'on the job' while 'doing the job'. Learning in the workplace enables students to learn about the context in which they will later practise.

Principles of work-based learning

WBL has powerful learning potential. A key underlying principle is that learning is inherent in everyday practice. The core condition for WBL is 'supported participation'. This involves the learner:

- **taking responsibility** for seeking out and engaging in learning experiences
- **being actively involved** in the context of the task being undertaken in the work situation
- **reflecting** on their learning experiences with mentors, supervisors, teachers and peers
- **interacting** with colleagues and other members of the healthcare team
- **receiving on-going feedback** from mentors, supervisors, teachers and peers.

Advantages of WBL

Learning on the job in the clinical environment offers a number of advantages:

- WBL focuses on real problems in the context of professional practice. Relevance, a key principle for effective learning as described in the FAIR model in Chapter 3, is a feature. It provides students/trainees with the satisfaction of doing a 'real job' in an authentic work setting rather than engaging in an academic exercise.
- WBL requires active participation and feedback – two other elements in the FAIR model. In WBL students learn more effectively through doing and through opportunities to practise, particularly when feedback is provided.
- WBL by its very nature can be designed to meet the needs of the learner – individualisation is the fourth component of the FAIR model.
- WBL offers a multiprofessional experience that can help students and trainees to work as a member of a team and develop their professional identity.
- Experience on the job can help students and trainees to make a career choice.
- Students' on-the-job experience, such as shadowing house officers in their final year as medical students, may prepare them for their subsequent posting after qualification. It helps them to become familiar with the work environment in the context of healthcare delivery. It may also help to enhance employment prospects for a particular post.

Implementation of WBL

Unfortunately the full potential of WBL is often not realised, and the expected learning outcomes are not achieved. The teacher can take several steps to optimise the potential of WBL in undergraduate education and postgraduate training:

- Plan the experience carefully, matching the learning experiences to the expected learning outcomes. What conditions are the student or trainee expected to see and what procedures are they expected to carry out? Unless planned carefully the school of experience is no school at all.
- Make the expectations explicit and draw up and agree a learning plan with the students/trainees.
- Monitor the learners' progress and provide constructive and timely feedback.
- Recognise the potential contributions of other members of the healthcare team to the students' and trainees' on-the-job experiences. The development of satisfactory relationships is an essential part of the exercise.
- Recognise the importance of the education environment. Students or trainees who are made to feel welcome are more likely to engage actively in the full range of learning opportunities provided and are more likely to play an active role within the team (Figure 19.1). The concept of the education environment is explored in Chapter 21.
- Make medical students an integral part of the patient's care. This may involve the student participating in ward rounds and in some aspects of the patient's management. A student's notes, for example, may become part of a patient's records, although this and other students' participation can present a legal challenge.
- The learner may benefit from a job aid that provides step-by-step guidelines for the tasks expected of them. This is particularly important when a task is

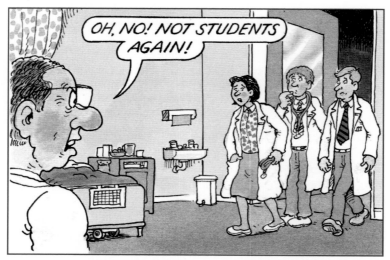

Figure 19.1 A negative attitude of the teacher can impact the students' learning

lengthy or complex, and when the consequence of error is high. The job aid may be presented in print format or electronically through a mobile device.

- A study guide can help the student or trainee to understand what is expected of them in the workplace and how they can obtain the maximum educational benefit from their experiences. The guide will help to relate these experiences to the other elements of the training programme and to relate theory to practice. Additional learning experiences such as the use of simulators that may enrich their experiences in the clinical setting are identified in the guide. The use of study guides is described in Chapter 15.

Problems and pitfalls of WBL

Problems and difficulties may be encountered when WBL is implemented:

- The learning may be opportunistic and based solely on the patients seen by the student or trainee. Some repetition of experiences is useful but unnecessary repetition should be avoided.
- The level of responsibility allocated to students or trainees in the delivery of the health care to the patients may present a problem. It is important that learners are not given tasks beyond their capabilities or authority.
- A conflict is sometimes perceived between the educational needs of the doctor in training and the service delivery demands. In WBL the relationship between the education and service components should be made explicit and the education integrated with the service delivery.
- The learner's progress needs to be carefully monitored and appropriate feedback provided, otherwise the learner is in danger of becoming like the golfer who continues to practise his mistakes but does not improve his game. Inappropriate or lack of feedback is a common criticism in WBL (Figure 19.2).

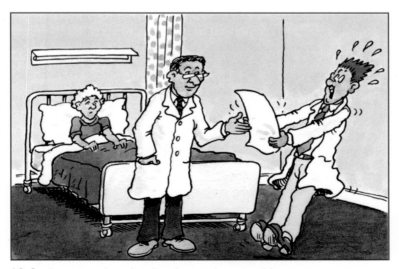

Figure 19.2 Inappropriate feedback may be a problem

The assessment of the students' progress and their achievement of the learning outcomes can be challenging. Non-traditional methods of assessment may be required and these are discussed in Section 5 on assessment.

* There may be funding implications for the medical school in undergraduate education where money follows the student. In postgraduate training there may be implications for the hospital if the employment of junior staff attracts higher insurance premiums.

Over to you

Reflect and react

1. Could the benefits of the apprenticeship model of education be captured in your training programme through work-based learning with the disadvantages avoided?
2. The work environment has powerful learning potential and can meet the criteria for effective and efficient learning. Is this potential fully achieved with your trainees?
3. Where are you on the continuum between hospital- and community-based education? Should you move more in the direction of community-based education?
4. Should longitudinal clinical clerkships be incorporated into your curriculum?

Explore further

Journal articles

Birden, H., Barker, J., Wilson, I., 2015. Effectiveness of a rural longitudinal integrated clerkship in preparing medical students for internship. Med. Teach. [Epub ahead of print].

Ellaway, R., Graves, L., Berry, S., et al., 2013. Twelve tips for designing and running longitudinal integrated clerkships. Med. Teach. 35, 989–995.

Hauer, K.E., Hirsh, D., Ma, I., et al., 2012. The role of role: learning in longitudinal integrated and traditional block clerkships. Med. Educ. 46, 698–710.
Students in a LIC feel greater competence in providing patient-centred care.

Hirsh, D.A., Holmboe, E.S., ten Cate, O., 2014. Time to trust: longitudinal integrated clerkships and entrustable professional activities. Acad. Med. 89, 201–204.
LICs and EPAs offer new possibilities for medical education.

Latessa, R., Beaty, N., Royal, K., et al., 2015. Academic outcomes of a community-based longitudinal integrated clerkships program. Med. Teach. 37, 862–867.
Students participating in a LIC outperformed students in a more traditional clinical rotation. Also useful reference list.

Mitchell, H.E., Harden, R.M., Laidlaw, J.M., 1998. Towards effective on-the-job learning: the development of a paediatric training guide. Med. Teach. 20, 91–98.
How WBL was implemented for junior doctors in a postgraduate paediatric training programme aided by a study guide.

Norris, T.E., Schaad, D.C., DeWitt, D., et al., 2009. Longitudinal integrated clerkships for medical students: an innovation adopted by medical schools in Australia, Canada, South Africa, and the United States. Acad. Med. 84, 902–907.

Strasser, R., Worley, P., Cristobal, F., et al., 2015. Putting communities in the driver's seat: the realities of community-engaged medical education. Acad. Med. 90 (11), 1466–1470.

Swanwick, T., 2005. Informal learning in postgraduate medical education: from cognitivism to 'culturism. Med. Educ. 39, 859–865.

Teherani, A., Irby, D.M., Loeser, H., 2013. Outcomes of different clerkship models: longitudinal integrated, hybrid, and block. Acad. Med. 88, 35–43.

The benefits to students increases with greater continuity.

Worley, P., Prideaux, D., Strasser, R., et al., 2006. Empirical evidence for symbiotic medical education: a comparative analysis of community and tertiary-based programmes. Med. Educ. 40, 109–116.

The examination performance of students on a rural general practice one-year programme was higher than that of their tertiary hospital-based peers.

Guides

Dornan, T., Littlewood, S., Margolis, S.A., et al., 2006. How can experience in clinical and community settings contribute to early medical education? A BEME systematic review. BEME Guide No. 6. Med. Teach. 28, 3–18.

Hudson, J.N., Poncelet, A.N., Weston, K.M., et al., 2016. Longitudinal integrated clerk-

ships. AMEE Guide No. 112. AMEE, Dundee.

Thistlethwaite, J.E., Bartle, E., Chong, A.A., et al., 2013. A review of longitudinal community and hospital placements in medical education. BEME Guide No. 26. Med. Teach. 35 (8).

Books

Calman, K., 2006. Medical Education: Past, Present and Future. Churchill Livingstone, London.

An interesting account of the history of medical education.

Websites

CLIC – The Consortium of Longitudinal Integrated Clerkships. <http://www.clicmeded.com>.

Schools who have or are considering adopting LICs in their curriculum.

The Network: Towards Unity for Health. <http://www.the-networktufh.org>.

A network of schools with a curriculum focus on community-based education.

Responding to information overload and building options into a core curriculum with threshold concepts

20

Alongside a core curriculum that provides the necessary breadth of study, options and electives provide an opportunity for students to study selected topics in more depth.

The problem of information overload

Information overload is one of the biggest problems facing students today. Advances in medicine and the so-called 'information explosion' have led to an increasing and potentially intolerable burden for the student. Curriculum committees are expected to pay attention to new topics and topics of particular concern such as team skills, professionalism, pain management, care of the dying, health education and personalised medicine. It has to be recognised, however, that the time available in a curriculum is finite and teachers cannot pack more and more into an already congested curriculum. They need to ensure that the time available is put to best use.

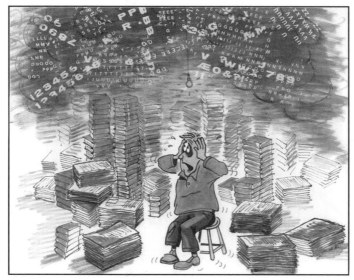

Figure 20.1 Information overload – a major problem facing medical education

Responding to the problem

In responding to the problem of information overload the teacher should:

- Recognise the need for students to move from simple fact memorisation to higher-level learning objectives, including searching, analysis and synthesis of information.
- Help students to develop expertise in accessing and retrieving information for themselves rather than teach students more than they can learn. A theme running through the book is the changing role of the teacher from information provider to someone who opens the door for learners to find information when they need it as a student and later as a doctor. Students need to be prepared for the future of practice where information is readily available to the doctor and the patient.
- Emphasise the core or essential learning required and the essential threshold concepts. Students must have significant knowledge from the core curriculum to be able to frame a good question and to ask for more information from appropriate sources (Friedman et al. 2016).
- Provide the students with the opportunity to study areas of their choosing in more depth during electives or student-selected components.

A core curriculum with options or student-selected components

Every curriculum should have both core curriculum elements and options, described as electives or student-selected components (SSCs).

A curriculum based on a core with options or electives, as recommended in 1993 by the UK General Medical Council in 'Tomorrow's Doctors', was a major development in curriculum planning. The precise place on the SPICES continuum between a standard and uniform curriculum and a curriculum entirely based on student-selected elements has to be determined by a school. The SSC is normally allocated 10–30% of the available curriculum time and 70–90% of the time allocated to the core. For the SSC this is equivalent to $\frac{1}{2}$ to $1\frac{1}{2}$ days per week or 3–9 weeks in an academic year.

Advantages of a core curriculum with SSCs

A core curriculum with SSCs embedded offers a number of advantages:

- The core curriculum highlights the essential learning requirements for all students and is consistent with an outcome-based education approach as described in Section 2.
- The establishment of a core curriculum helps to counter the danger that increasing specialisation in medicine will dominate the curriculum.
- A description of the core curriculum helps to determine the equivalence of training in different schools or countries and facilitates the mobility of doctors.

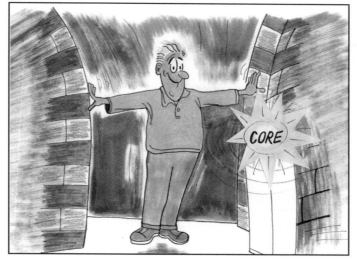

Figure 20.2   Core learning outcomes should be highlighted

- The core curriculum provides a standard against which students can be assessed.
- Students have the opportunity to cover the breadth of knowledge in the core element of the curriculum while at the same time they are able to study in depth selected subjects of their choosing.
- Special study modules may be offered in subjects not normally addressed in the curriculum.
- Experience of a subject during an SSC may help students with regard to their career choice.
- Completion of a series of SSCs in a subject may count towards postgraduate training in that area and shorten the duration of training. It is not the norm at present, but may be more widely recognised in the future.
- Teachers value interacting in SSCs with an enthusiastic group of students who have a special interest in their subject and who might be the researchers or teachers of the future.

Specification of a core curriculum

The specification of the core curriculum should be the responsibility of all the stakeholders, including the clinicians and basic scientists. It should not be left to each discipline or specialty to specify the core curriculum in their area. The content can be determined as described in Chapter 9.

Topics merit inclusion in a core curriculum if they are:

- common in clinical practice
- representative of a serious or life-threatening situation in clinical practice

- an important prerequisite for other learning and illustrate an important principle.

The core curriculum is reflected in:

- the statement of learning outcomes, as described in Section 2
- problems presented in a PBL curriculum
- patient presentations used as a framework for the curriculum
- learning opportunities provided for the students
- the assessment of the students.

Threshold concepts

Threshold concepts are a relatively new idea in medical education and have not been widely researched or applied. Given the problem of information overload, however, it is an approach that merits further consideration. Threshold concepts were identified in a report by the Open University in the UK as one of the new pedagogies with the potential to bring about major shifts in educational practice (Sharples et al. 2014).

A consideration of threshold concepts helps teachers to make decisions about what learners need to understand relating to a topic if they are to master it. This has been described as the portal or gateway giving students access to a new way of thinking. For the student they are the 'eureka' moments in learning that open up previously inaccessible ways of understanding something (Meyer et al. 2010).

Key characteristics

Meyer et al. (2010) describe the key characteristics of a threshold concept. For better understanding, we have used a gardening analogy:

- They are *transformative*, bringing about a significant new perception of a subject. A threshold concept in gardening is that plants require different amounts of water for their cultivation. If this concept is ignored and all plants are provided with the same amount of water some plants will fail to grow.
- They are *integrative*, exploring connections that may have been previously hidden. In the gardening analogy the understanding of water requirements leads to a better understanding of soil requirements.
- They are *irreversible* and unlikely to be forgotten or unlearned – only through considerable effort. Once the principle is learned that plants require different amounts of water, this is unlikely to be forgotten. The student may forget, however, how they mastered the concept and the teacher may forget their own struggles mastering the concept.
- They are *troublesome* in the sense that they may be counterintuitive or seemingly incoherent. Common sense may in fact inhibit mastery of a threshold concept. That plants with similar appearances have different water

requirements is not obvious and those who previously thought that plants need similar amounts of water may have difficulty in changing their beliefs.

The importance of threshold concepts

There is competition for time and space in the curriculum and a consideration of threshold concepts can contribute to decisions about what to include. Failure to grasp the required threshold concepts may prevent a student from progressing. My (RMH) grand-daughter successfully coached a fellow student who had repeatedly failed the maths examination at school and this had prevented his progression to the next class. She found that the student lacked an understanding of a few basic principles in maths. Once this was recognised and the principles mastered, the student went on to perform well in maths examinations and progressed normally.

In a spiral curriculum as described in Chapter 14, it is helpful to identify the threshold concepts that are required at each stage of the curriculum and necessary as prior knowledge for the next phase.

Electives/SSCs

The concept of electives is not new. They are often undertaken overseas, and provide students with an international focus and opportunity to experience different cultures. What is different with the 'core and option' curriculum concept is that the options or SSCs can be varied, are closely integrated into the curriculum and contribute to the core curriculum outcomes. Learning outcomes for the elective curriculum may be content-independent and embrace higher-order competencies such as independent learning, self-assessment and professionalism. It is through the options that students may have the greatest opportunity to direct their own learning and to learn to assess their own progress.

Choice of SSC topics

A wide range of topics can be addressed in SSCs. These include:

- A more in-depth study of subjects included in the core curriculum. With a reduction in time allocated to basic sciences in the curriculum, students with an interest in the area have an opportunity to study anatomy or another basic science in more depth.
- Special aspects of clinical practice such as plastic surgery not covered in the curriculum.
- Topics unrelated to medicine but of possible relevance to a doctor's future career, for example the study of a foreign language or business studies.
- Medical education and teaching skills. This is now offered as an option in a number of schools. We have seen students make useful contributions to the curriculum and generate useful learning resource material during an SSC.
- Interprofessional experiences, for example working as a member of an interprofessional team or shadowing a nurse. The latter proved a popular SSC in Dundee but mainly for female students.

- Research, which may be clinical, laboratory-based or educational.

Students may choose from a list of options provided by the medical school or identify their own area for further study which is approved by the school.

Assessment of SSCs

The assessment of SSCs should be transparent and related to the contribution the SSC makes to the learning outcomes for the course. The assessment of students' performance in SSCs must be integrated with their overall programme of assessment. The SSC assessment should be used to determine the student's progress alongside their performance in the core curriculum

A range of methods may be used. Portfolio assessment, as described in Chapter 33, offers a number of advantages. Problems relating to fairness and equivalence need to be addressed, given the varying nature of different electives.

Integration of SSCs with the core

SSCs can be integrated in the timetable with the core curriculum in different ways:

- **Sequential.** A block of core teaching, for example 8 weeks, is followed by a 2-week SSC option. This allows the student to explore the subject of the preceding block in more detail, or to study an unrelated subject.
- **Intermittent.** Blocks of time, for example 4–10 weeks, are allocated for SSCs at set times in the curriculum.
- **Concurrent.** The SSC topic is scheduled for half or one day per week alongside the core but on a topic not necessarily related to the core.
- **Integrated.** The SSC is integrated within the core topic programme allowing the student to study different aspects of the core in more depth. One option for an endocrinology course offered at Dundee was for the student to choose between exploring in more detail the laboratory investigation of endocrine disease, endocrine surgery or the management of endocrine problems in the community.

Over to you

Reflect and react

1. Whether you are working in undergraduate or postgraduate training, has the appropriate balance between the core curriculum and electives or SSCs been achieved in your programme? Has the core curriculum been specified so as to leave time for electives or SSCs?
2. Have threshold concepts been considered for your course, and if not should they be?
3. Are the learning outcomes for the SSCs clear to the students and supervisors, and are they assessed appropriately?
4. Is a sufficient choice of SSCs available to students, and are they given sufficient guidance to make their choice?

Explore further

Journal articles

Cousin, G., 2006. An introduction to threshold concepts. Planet 17, 4–5.
The development of the idea of threshold concepts.

Friedman, C.P., Donaldson, K.M., Vantsevich, A.V., 2016. Educating medical students in the era of ubiquitous information. Med. Teach. Epub ahead of print.
The competencies students need to acquire to seek and analyse available information.

Kinchin, I.M., Cabot, L.B., Kobus, M., Woolford, M., 2011. Threshold concepts in dental education. Eur. J. Dent. Educ. 15, 210–215.
An example of the use of threshold concepts in dental education.

Law, I.R., Worley, P.S., Langham, F.J., 2013. International medical electives undertaken by Australian medical students: current trends and future directions. Med. J. Aust. 198, 324–326.

Neve, H., Wearn, A., Collett, T., 2015. What are threshold concepts and how can they inform medical education? Med. Teach. Epub ahead of print.

Guides

Harden, R.M., Davis, M., 2001. The core curriculum with options or special study modules. AMEE Education Guide No. 5. Med. Teach. 23, 231–244.

Lumb, A., Murdoch-Eaton, D., 2014. Electives in undergraduate medical education: AMEE Guide No. 88. Med. Teach. 36, 557–572.

Riley, S.C., 2009. Student selected components. AMEE Guide No. 46. Med. Teach. 31, 885–894.

Reports

Sharples, M., Adams, A., Ferguson, R., et al., 2014. Innovating Pedagogy 2014: Open University Innovation Report 3. The Open University Press, Milton Keynes.

Books

Meyer, J.H.F., Land, R., Baillie, C. (Eds.), 2010. Threshold concepts and transformational learning. Sense Publishers, Rotterdam, The Netherlands.
A definitive text on threshold concepts.

Recognising the importance of the education environment 21

This neglected area is now recognised as being a substantial and very real element that influences students' learning. Tools are available to assess the education environment.

What is the learning environment

We can read the curriculum documents, we can inspect the expected learning outcomes and we can experience a wide range of teaching approaches, but we may know little about the student's experience in the education programme. Key to this, suggests Genn (2001), is the atmosphere or climate experienced by the student in the school – what is valued, what is recognised and what is encouraged. He describes the education climate as the soul and heart of the medical school. It is the education environment that determines the students' behaviour, their achievements and their satisfaction. McAleer and Roff (2013) likened it to the climate or environment in the meteorological context and suggested that we cannot hope to maximise the education output if we do not foster a nurturing climate.

Contributing to the learning environment in a medical school or a postgraduate programme and influencing the students' or trainees' learning, positively or negatively, are:

- how students are taught and the education strategies adopted
- what they are taught
- how they are assessed
- the types of clinical experiences offered
- the books and resources available online or in the library
- the values expressed by their teachers
- physical factors such as lecture theatre seating, heating, cooling and levels of noise.

The education climate is important

The establishment of an appropriate climate is almost certainly the most important single task for a medical teacher. It is the educational climate that ultimately

153

determines a student's behaviour – what and how they learn. Genn and others have highlighted that while the education climate may seem rather intangible, unreal and insubstantial, its effects are pervasive, substantial, very real and influential. The climate, it has been suggested, is like a mist – you cannot stay long in the mist before being thoroughly soaked. The climate includes the type of things that are rewarded, encouraged and emphasised, and the style of life that is valued in the school or training programme.

A study of the learning environment can help to answer questions such as:

- Is collaboration or competition between students encouraged?
- Is the student encouraged to ask questions and think creatively or to participate passively and follow the rules?
- Is the curriculum about meeting the needs of the learner or the needs of the teacher?
- Does the curriculum challenge and stretch students or require only minimum competence?
- Is the environment a trusting one where the teacher is supportive and tolerant of mistakes or is the teacher viewed with suspicion as the 'enemy' of the student?

Without an examination of the education environment these questions go unanswered. Genn (2001) suggests, 'If we wish to describe, assess, or otherwise "get a handle on" the curriculum in a medical school, we need to consider the environment, educational and organisational, associated with the curriculum and the medical school.'

In postgraduate training, particular concerns have related to poor supervision, variable and unpredictable teaching, lack of continuity, the provision of feedback that is not constructive, and an emphasis on service requirements rather than educational requirements. These can all be related to the existing education environment.

Suggestions that students become more cynical and less empathetic as they progress through the medical curriculum are a cause of concern. The problem may rest, at least in part, with the education environment. Too often this is task-orientated with the emphasis on the presentation by an expert scientist or clinician. They know the answers and procedures while the social-emotional orientation concerning the development of a caring helper of sick people is neglected. An appropriate education environment should encourage the development of abilities to empathise and identify with patients and their predicaments.

The need for a fundamental review of medical education was proposed by the Global Independent Commission on Education of Health Professionals for the 21st Century published in *The Lancet* in December 2010. The recommendations proposed far-reaching changes to learning outcomes and to methods of teaching, learning and assessment, and addressed issues relating to teamwork, interprofessional collaboration, international dimensions and individualised learning. One could argue that key to the implementation of these changes is the development of a supportive education environment.

Aspects of the education environment

The medical education environment is extraordinarily complex. The different dimensions are sometimes referred to as orientations. Some aspects or orientations of the environment that merit consideration are listed here. It is not a comprehensive list but it provides examples of the various orientations.

Collaborative or competitive orientation

It is a paradox that teamwork and collaboration are identified as important learning outcomes in medical training and the interprofessional team is recognised, but the training programme with which our students and trainees engage fosters competition rather than collaboration. Students are recognised and rewarded on the basis of their individual performance and not on their performance as a member of a team or group.

For a collaborative education environment, students need to develop a feeling of 'belonging' in the group or team. They should be encouraged to work with their colleagues and participate as part of a ward team in clinical attachments. In a PBL curriculum and in team-based learning the team process is valued.

Student or teacher orientation

The education environment may be one in which the teacher is more valued than the student. In a student-centred environment it is the learner who is valued. Their interests, impact on the curriculum, and independence and autonomy are encouraged, as discussed in Chapter 15.

Supportive or punitive orientation

Students or trainees in the past have been left to their own devices to deal with academic or personal problems. Some students have found the teaching threatening or intimidating, especially if they have been humiliated or harassed. This type of environment has been seen as helping to toughen up the student, with survival viewed as some sort of rite of passage. Learners were encouraged to cover up any difficulties experienced or refrain from divulging gaps in their knowledge. Fortunately the climate has changed. Students are encouraged to assess their own progress and identify any difficulties they might have with the assurance that support and counselling are available. In a supportive education environment, learners are free to experiment, voice their concerns, identify their lack of knowledge and stretch their limits.

Community or hospital orientation

Medical education has been criticised as having as its base an ivory tower academic centre, distant from the realities of the day-to-day practice of family medicine in the community. Professors and specialists with international recognition are the role models for the students. It is perhaps not surprising that, in the past, a career in general practice or in a rural community was frowned on by students as being a 'second best' choice. Fortunately this tension has now been recognised and there is a greater emphasis, as described in Chapter 19, on students learning in the community and in the rural setting with some medical schools established in a rural location.

Research or teaching orientation

The teaching and learning programme may be conducted in the context of an environment where research is valued and rewarded, and where teaching is seen as an activity that encroaches on writing research papers or proposals for funding. Some medical schools are trying to redress the balance by recognising the scholarship of teaching as a criterion for appointments and promotions. Newly appointed faculty members may be expected to demonstrate, or acquire through a staff development programme, expertise in teaching. Excellence in education in a medical school is now recognised by the ASPIRE-to-excellence initiative (http://www.aspire-to-excellence.org).

The effects of the environment

The educational climate may manifest itself in a number of ways:

- The education environment makes a unique and notable contribution to the prediction of student achievement and success.
- The motivation of the learner is influenced by the education environment in which he or she is studying.
- The education environment along with other factors can have a significant impact on career choice. Preference for a career as a surgeon in an academic centre, or for a career as a general practitioner in a rural community, may be attributed to the training programme's education environment.
- Staff may be more inclined to stay in a post if an institution has a 'good' education environment. It is easier to attract new staff to such an institution.

Assessment of the education environment

One reason why the education environment was ignored in the past was the lack of a suitable instrument or tool to measure it. A number of validated instruments are now available for use in different settings. McAleer and Roff (2013) described thirty such tools and provided a useful summary of them. Frequently used are the Dundee Ready Education Environment Measure (DREEM) and the Postgraduate Hospital Education Environment Measure (PHEEM). The educational environment can be assessed using qualitative as well as quantitative approaches. A qualitative approach involves collecting data using a survey instrument with open-ended questions such as 'What do you most like about your training programme?', or by eliciting feedback from focus groups. With quantitative instruments students are asked to reply to a series of questions, with each question relating to one aspect or dimension of the education environment.

DREEM has five subscales, as described in Appendix 8:

- Students' perceptions of learning
- Students' perceptions of teachers
- Students' academic self-perceptions
- Students' perceptions of atmosphere
- Students' social self-perceptions

DREEM contains fifty statements that cover these dimensions. A 5-point scale is used to score each item from 0 for 'strongly disagree' to 4 for 'strongly agree'. There is a maximum score of 200, indicating the ideal education environment as perceived by the student. Excellence is indicated by a score of 151–200.

Instruments have been developed to assess the education environment in postgraduate education (PHEEM), in the anaesthetic theatre (ATEEM) and in the surgery theatre (STEEM) (Roff, 2005).

The use of environment measures

Measurements of the education environment can be used to:

- establish the profile for an institution and gain a holistic view of the curriculum
- understand students' perceptions of the education environment they have experienced and compare it with their perception of the ideal environment
- compare the perceptions of the different stakeholders including staff, students and managers
- compare the environment as it exists in different departments or attachments within a school and at different phases of the training programme
- provide the medical school or postgraduate body, as a 'learning organisation', with an indication of what may be lacking in their programme and where change may be necessary, while at the same time nurturing aspects where no change is required
- assess the effect of a change made in the curriculum, comparing the education environment before and after the change
- compare the environment of different medical schools or geographical settings.

Over to you

Reflect and react

1. The education climate or environment is a key factor in the success of an undergraduate or postgraduate education programme. Think about what type of learning environment you would wish to have as a student and how this compares with the learning environment that exists in your training programme.

RECOGNISING THE IMPORTANCE OF THE EDUCATION ENVIRONMENT

2. Measurement of the education environment provides valuable information relating to curriculum planning and evaluation. If information is not already available, measure the education environment in your teaching situation using one of the tools available. On the basis of the results, think about how the programme could be improved.

3. Reflect on how your own teaching and attitudes contribute to the education environment as perceived by students or trainees.

Explore further

Journal articles

Colbert-Getz, J.M., Kim, S., Goode, V.H., 2014. Assessing medical students' and residents' perceptions of the learning environment: exploring validity evidence for the interpretation of scores from existing tools. Acad. Med. 89, 1687–1693.

Frenk, J., Chen, L., Bhutta, Z.A., et al., 2010. Health professionals for a new century: transforming education to strengthen health systems in an interdependent world. Lancet 376, 1923–1958.

An authoritative report on the changes needed in medical education.

Holt, M.C., Roff, S., 2004. Development and validation of the anaesthetic theatre educational environment measure (ATEEM). Med. Teach. 26, 553–558.

Miles, S., Swift, L., Leinster, S.J., 2012. The Dundee Ready Education Environment Measure (DREEM): a review of its adoption and use. Med. Teach. 34, e620–e634.

Roff, S., 2005. Education environment: a bibliography. Med. Teach. 27, 353–357.

A list of more than 100 relevant articles.

Roff, S., McAleer, S., Harden, R.M., et al., 1997. Development and validation of the Dundee Ready Education Environment Measure (DREEM). Med. Teach. 19, 295–299.

The first description of this important inventory.

Roff, S., McAleer, S., Skinner, A., 2005. Development and validation of an instrument to measure the postgraduate clinical learning and teaching educational environment for hospital-based junior doctors in the UK. Med. Teach. 27, 327–331.

A description of the development of the Postgraduate Hospital Educational Environment Measure (PHEEM).

Shobhana, N., Wall, D., Jones, E., 2006. Can STEEM be used to measure the educational environment within the operating theatre for undergraduate medical students? Med. Teach. 28, 642–647.

Shochet, R.B., Colbert-Getz, J.M., Wright, S.M., 2015. The Johns Hopkins learning environment scale: measuring medical students' perceptions of the process supporting professional formation. Acad. Med. 90, 810–818.

Guides

Genn, J.M., 2001. Curriculum, environment, climate, quality and change in medical education – a unifying perspective. AMEE Medical Education Guide No. 23. Med. Teach. 23, 445–454.

A key text on the subject that merits careful reading.

Books

McAleer, S., Roff, S., 2013. Educational environment. In: Dent, J.A., Harden, R.M. (Eds.), A Practical Guide for Medical Teachers, fourth ed. Elsevier, London (Chapter 48).

A review of the concept and how the educational environment can be measured.

A clear picture of how learning outcomes, teaching methods and student assessment link together is crucial not only for the teacher but also for the student. A curriculum map is needed.

The need for a curriculum map

Planning a curriculum, as described in the earlier chapters, is a complex matter involving learning outcomes, content, a timetable, the programme of teaching and learning opportunities and assessment. In planning and designing a curriculum an aspect that has been relatively neglected is how the details of the curriculum will be communicated to all of the stakeholders. How do teachers and students know what is covered and where it is addressed? How do students know what learning opportunities are available to assist them in mastering the learning outcomes? How does assessment relate to the teaching programme and are there gaps between what is taught and what is assessed? Unfortunately students and trainees may perceive a curriculum or educational programme as a 'magical mystery tour' with the answers to these questions uncertain. They are not quite sure what lies ahead, or even about their destination, apart from the fact that they will end up with a qualification if they complete the course satisfactorily. The challenge is to ensure that staff and students are well informed about the curriculum and this can be done using curriculum mapping.

What is a curriculum map?

A curriculum map is a visual representation of a curriculum that shows the big picture and how the different elements are related and linked together. It presents the curriculum as a sophisticated blend of educational strategies, course content, learning outcomes, educational experiences, assessment and programme of courses. Basically it provides information about what is taught, how it is taught, when it is taught, where it is taught and how the learning is assessed. It should be a key feature of any curriculum and it can even be thought of as the glue that holds the curriculum together.

Curriculum mapping is on today's agenda

There are a number of reasons why a curriculum map is now an essential element in planning and implementing a curriculum:

- **Outcome-based education.** The map makes explicit the expected learning outcomes for the different courses and learning experiences provided.
- **Student-centred learning.** The map of the curriculum helps the students to take responsibility for their own learning, to appreciate what they are studying and the part it plays in the bigger picture, and how they can tailor the learning experiences to their personal needs.
- **Clinical presentations, problem-based and integrated learning.** A map can help students to understand and visualise the relationship between the clinical presentations or tasks used as a framework for the curriculum, the learning outcomes and the learning opportunities illustrated in the curriculum cube described in Chapter 16. It helps to clarify the learning outcomes in PBL and integrated teaching programmes and the contributors from the different disciplines.
- **Interprofessional education.** Described in a map are the common elements and the differences in the curriculum between medicine and other professions. This facilitates the planning of interprofessional activities.
- **Integration of assessment and teaching.** The relationship between teaching and assessment is demonstrated in the map in keeping with the move described in Section 5 towards 'assessment-for-learning'.
- **Distributed learning.** A map helps to ensure uniformity in the curriculum where this is delivered by a medical school on two or more sites.
- **Student mobility.** The transparency of the learning programme implicit in a curriculum map allows students' work to be recognised if they transfer to a different location. As envisaged in the Bologna process, on completion of the first cycle a student may move to complete the second cycle of their medical studies in another school.
- **The continuum of education.** A curriculum map assists the seamless transition between the different phases of undergraduate, postgraduate and continuing education and what is addressed in each phase.
- **Curriculum evaluation.** The curriculum map is a valuable tool for both internal and external assessment of the education programme, including more formal accreditation and review by the public.
- **Changes in medicine.** A curriculum should be dynamic and not static in order that it can accommodate advances in medical practice. New subjects integrated into the curriculum are highlighted in the map. At the same time any redundancies and duplications in the curriculum can be recognised.

Curriculum mapping can be seen in terms of the six 'C's' (Figure 22.1).

Potential users of the curriculum map

The curriculum map may be of value to:

- **Teachers**. The map provides an overview of the curriculum programme in its entirety so that teachers can appreciate the place of their course within the curriculum and identify their own roles and responsibilities. Students or

Curriculum planning, implementation and evaluation

Competency-based education

Communicating about the curriculum

Continuum of education across undergraduate, postgraduate and continuing education

Collaboration with all of the stakeholders including the other healthcare professions

Changes in the learning outcomes and the educational programme

Figure 22.1 The 6 Cs of curriculum mapping

trainees frequently complain that incorrect assumptions are made by staff about the topics covered elsewhere in the curriculum.

- **Curriculum planners**. The map provides a tool to assist the planner to evaluate the curriculum and keep it up to date. The map can be used to study whether what it is assumed the students are learning (the 'declared curriculum'), the curriculum that is presented (the 'delivered curriculum') and what the students actually learn (the 'learned curriculum') are aligned.
- **Students**. The curriculum map together with the statement of expected learning outcomes and a study guide provide students with information that helps them to plan their programme of work and to assess their progress.
- **Administrators and support staff**. A curriculum map assists staff with the identification of resources necessary to implement the curriculum, including staff, equipment and accommodation. It may also help to determine the contributions made by academic departments or individual members of staff to the curriculum and allow this to be recognised and rewarded.
- **Educational researchers**. There is a growing interest in research in medical education. The curriculum map is a useful tool for research into the existing curriculum or into changes made with regard to the teaching and assessment programme.
- **Accrediting bodies**. The map may help to provide evidence that the medical school or postgraduate programme meets the expected requirements set out by accreditors. In the UK, the General Medical Council when accrediting a school expects to see a curriculum map. The curriculum map is used to obtain an outline of the course, as a search tool to enquire about the curriculum and to check spiralling of the curriculum, for omissions and excesses and that the institution is adhering to the GMC recommendations in *Tomorrow's Doctors*.

Preparing a curriculum map

Just for a moment put yourself in a different context. You are faced with planning a one-year's excursion to a part of the world with which you are unfamiliar. The first thing you need to inform your travel around the region is a map. This will show the different destinations and how each is located one to the other, the different transport options including roads, railways and airports, and the sites of objects of interest such as castles, lakes, etc. In much the same way a map of the curriculum includes:

- the expected learning outcomes
- the content, themes or topics addressed
- the learning experiences and resources available
- the assessment
- the courses and modules studied
- the timetable schedule.

The strength of the map lies in the links between these elements. For example, the learning outcomes, the learning experiences and the assessment are specified for each course or elements within a course or module. The maximum benefit is achieved through this multi-dimensionality with the ability to examine the curriculum from the perspective of any one element or window. For example, where in the curriculum is the communication skills learning outcome addressed? From the assessment perspective, where is professionalism evaluated? What is the role of the clinical skills centre in the training programme?

Curriculum mapping has been limited by problems associated with storing, manipulating and updating the large amounts of information that cannot be viewed easily from different perspectives. The availability of electronic tools, including multi-relational databases, has given the concept of curriculum mapping a new impetus. Many schools that have developed a curriculum map have produced their own mapping programme. Curriculum mapping tools available include Ilios, a tool developed by a consortium of US medical schools (https://www.iliosproject.org) and a product from Innovative Technology.

A Google search for 'curriculum mapping medical schools' demonstrates that medical schools have adopted different approaches to the preparation of a curriculum map. The basis for a curriculum map may be a list of the courses or modules delivered over a period of time. To this can be added information about the learning outcomes, the learning experiences and the assessment of the course. It may be helpful in the first instance in the preparation of a map to think about a series of two-dimensional matrices. For each learning opportunity event timetabled, for example, the learning outcomes and the student assessment are specified.

Teachers should be actively involved in the construction and updating of a curriculum map and in its application to their own teaching – 'curriculum mapping is not a spectator sport. It demands teachers' ongoing preparation and active participation' (Hale 2008).

Over to you

Reflect and react

1. The curriculum map highlights that the curriculum is greater than the sum of the parts, demonstrating the integration of the different elements. Think about how information relating to your curriculum is communicated to the students or trainees. To what extent is a map of the curriculum available that highlights for each part of the programme the learning outcomes, the learning opportunities and resources and the assessment procedures?

2. There has been renewed interest in curriculum mapping with input from educationalists, technologists, teachers, content experts, curriculum managers and students. The investment of time in the production of a map for the curriculum can be rewarding and result in a much more powerful teaching and learning experience. Can you set some time aside to work on this with your colleagues?

Explore further

Journal articles

Al-Eraky, M.M., 2012. Curriculum navigator: aspiring towards a comprehensive package for curriculum planning. Med. Teach. 34, 724–732.

A conceptual framework for exploring the curriculum.

Hege, I., Nowak, D., Kolb, S., et al., 2010. Developing and analysing a curriculum map in Occupational- and Environmental medicine. BMC Med. Educ. 10, 60.

Ross, N., Davies, D., 1999. Outcome-based learning and the electronic curriculum at Birmingham Medical School. Med. Teach. 21, 26–31.

West, C.A., Graham, L., 2015. Maps, gaps, and modules. Med. Sci. Educ. 25, 213–214.

Experience in Texas using a curriculum map.

Guides

Harden, R.M., 2001. Curriculum mapping: a tool for transparent and authentic teaching and learning. AMEE Guide No. 21. Med. Teach. 23, 123–137.

Books

Hale, J.A., 2008. A Guide to Curriculum Mapping: Planning, Implementing, and Sustaining the Process. Corwin Press, Thousand Oaks, CA.

Jacobs, H.H. (Ed.), 2004. Getting Results with Curriculum Mapping. ASCD, Alexandria, VA.

A wide range of perspectives and advice on curriculum mapping in schools.

Website

Heidi, H.J., 2012. What is curriculum mapping? [Video file.] <http://www.youtube.com/watch?v=8etEUVzo2GE> YouTube, April 3rd.

An account of curriculum mapping by an innovator in the field.

SECTION 4
Styles of Teaching

'There can be no single way to study or best way to teach.'
Noel Entwistle. *Styles of Learning and Teaching*, 1981

- Choose the most appropriate method from the rich menu of learning opportunities available and use it to maximum effect
- Lectures can make a valuable contribution to the education programme. Careful consideration needs to be given to the reason for their use and how they are delivered. A 'flipped classroom' may be useful
- Small group teaching has a part to play if used appropriately. The teacher's role is different from their role in a lecture
- Students and trainees should be given more responsibility for their own learning. The learner may require support and direction
- Lack of planning and poor supervision coupled with inadequate feedback to students often blights clinical teaching
- Simulated patients, manikins, models and computer simulations complement experience with 'real' patients and have a place in a training programme
- The Internet and resources available online have revolutionised medical education. They can make a significant contribution to the education programme
- Students learning from each other is effective. This can be informal or incorporated into scheduled activities

The lecture and teaching with large groups 23

Lectures can make a valuable contribution to the education pro-gramme. Careful consideration needs to be given to the reasons for their use and how they are delivered.

The use of lectures

Of all the approaches to teaching, the lecture is perhaps the method most widely adopted. It is estimated that the average medical student sits through some 1800 lectures in the course of their studies. Most will be quickly forgotten: a few may be memorable. Despite much criticism, the lecture has stood the test of time. It has a lot to offer and it should not be tossed aside as being ineffective and as a result excluded from the teacher's toolkit as described in Chapter 13.

Brown and Manogue (2001) describe lectures as an economical and efficient method of conveying information to large groups of students. The lecture can provide an entrée into a difficult topic, it can offer different perspectives on a subject, it can communicate relevant personal, clinical or laboratory experience, and it can deliver a research-based view where teaching is immersed in a research-intensive university.

The way lectures are being used, however, is changing, with greater engagement of students during the lecture and recordings of lectures being made available to students. In the 'flipped classroom' model there is a fundamental change in the nature of the use made of the time previously allocated to a formal lecture.

Problems with lectures

Problems attributed to the lecture may be the result of a 'bad lecturer' or the inappropriate use of the lecture. Common criticisms of lectures (Figure 23.1) include:

- The lecture is a passive learning experience with a failure to engage students in their own learning.
- Much of what is covered can be learned better from reading a book or engaging in an online programme.

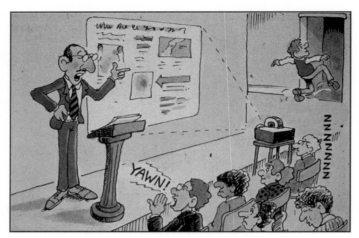

Figure 23.1 The lecture has been much criticised

- The lecture is badly presented and difficult to follow, with the visuals overloaded with information.
- The content of the lecture is inappropriate for the audience and is irrelevant, too advanced or too simple.

When to use lectures

Lectures, if used properly, offer a number of advantages:

- The lecturer can meet simultaneously with a large group of students and convey his or her passion and enthusiasm for a subject.
- The lecture can serve as an introduction to a difficult topic and provide the students with a framework for their further studies.
- Dealing with a controversial area, the lecture can provide different perspectives and at the same time relate the topic to the local context.
- In an advancing area of knowledge, the lecture can provide up-to-date information and highlight the contributions of research in an area.
- The lecture can be used to provoke thought and discussion and to encourage the student to reflect on the topic.
- The lecture can include a practical demonstration, for example with a cardiac simulator or a patient introduced to illustrate a point (with the agreement of the patient).
- The lecture can provide the students with guidelines about their further study of the topic and can introduce the resources and other learning opportunities available.

Delivering a good lecture

Lecturing can be a daunting task for some teachers, who feel ill at ease when asked to perform in front of a large audience of students. Much of the stress can be alleviated with good planning and preparation.

Get some facts in advance

Before concentrating on the content of the lecture, first do some fact finding:

- Study the learning outcomes for the course. Based on these, consider how the lecture fits into the curriculum.
- Find out what the students already know about the subject of the lecture.
- Establish whether the lecture is one of a series of lectures on the subject and, if so, what the other lectures cover.
- Find out about the venue and the equipment to be used.

Think about the content and structure

Plan in advance the content and structure of the lecture:

- Plan the content for a lecture the students will wish to hear rather than the lecture you would like to give.
- Create a title for the lecture. It is sometimes easier to get started with the content if you first think of a title as it helps to structure your thoughts. It is more likely to interest students if the title is in the form of a question.
- Consider how you wish to structure the lecture. Two commonly used approaches are the classical method, where the lecture content is divided up into broad areas which are then subdivided, and the problem-centred approach, where a problem or case study is presented and solutions are discussed. This chapter focuses on the classical approach although most of the tips given apply to both approaches.
- Lecturing styles vary considerably, so you must choose the style you feel most comfortable with and which suits your personality.

The introduction to the lecture

It is worth spending some time preparing your introduction. The first few minutes of the lecture are the most valuable. Try to instantly capture the attention of the audience and highlight why the content of the lecture is important. An engaging start to a lecture might include a press cutting of a case where an error has been made in the management of a patient. It could be an illustration of a patient where an understanding of the pathophysiology proved valuable in the patient's management. You might use an interesting statistic highlighting the importance of the topic. Robert Cialdini is quoted as saying at the beginning of a lecture 'Here's a set of events unexplainable by common sense, and I promise you'll be able to solve this mystery at the end of the class.'

Don't keep the student in the dark about the content of the lecture. Tell the student what you are going to tell them, then tell them and finally tell them what you have told them. Advance organisers can help. These are signposts that help to guide the student through the content as you have structured it. For example, 'we will look in turn at six features of ...' or 'first we will look at ... then at ... and finally at ...'.

Visual aids

Visual aids help to reinforce and emphasise important points in a lecture and to explain difficult concepts or principles. They also help to vary the pace of the lecture and to maintain the student's interest. Video clips can be used to introduce case studies. Check for typographical errors on text visuals as spelling mistakes damage your credibility. Also make sure that students at the back of the lecture theatre will be able to read the text or captions on your visuals. It is amazing how many teachers fail to do this.

PowerPoint is an application designed to help the speaker or lecturer assemble professional-looking slides and is widely used in oral presentations. The result sadly is often an unending stream of slides with bullet lists, animations that obscure rather than clarify the point and cartoons that distract from rather than convey the message. A host of sites are available on the Web that provide practical advice on PowerPoint presentations and can help you to avoid 'death by PowerPoint' (Harden 2008).

Visual aids are a tool to help the teacher get a message across to students in the most effective way. The lecturer, not the PowerPoint slides, should be the star of the occasion. The text on slides should complement what is being said, not replace it.

Engaging the audience

There are a number of strategies that can be adopted to transform your presentation from a passive to an engaging and active experience for the student. These include:

- Introduce questions on the subject at various stages during the lecture, with a number of alternative answers presented. Students are asked to respond using an electronic response system, or coloured cards can be used with a different colour corresponding to each answer. Electronic response systems use either devices or 'clickers' which allow each student to respond to multiple choice questions, usually incorporated into a PowerPoint presentation or an app which enables students to respond by web, text and Twitter. Students go to a URL and questions are posted to that URL. A range of products are available in both categories.
- Incorporate mini brainstorming sessions during the lecture where groups of three, four or five students next to each other are encouraged to discuss a topic. Some groups are asked to report back to the whole class. Alternatively the groups may answer and respond to a multiple choice question using cards or an audience response system. This is a key activity in team-based learning.
- Introduce or build your presentation around a case study or patient management problem, involving the class as the problem develops.

The close of the lecture

The end of the lecture is almost as important as the introduction. Summarise the main concepts or messages you wish to convey and prepare the students for any further lectures that may follow in the series. Try also to leave students with something to think about following the lecture, which may stimulate a discussion with their colleagues.

Handouts

A printed or digital summary of the lecture can provide the student with the framework and also the essential messages you wish to convey. It can be designed in such a way that students are encouraged to personalise it with their own notes as the lecture proceeds. Handouts may be valuable for revision purposes. Some lecturers use copies of their PowerPoint presentation as handouts but this is less satisfactory than handouts designed specifically for the purpose. If you want to encourage students to take notes during the lecture, make sure that you leave sufficient time for this activity.

Students' presence and behaviour at lectures

There has been an increasing trend for medical schools to video lectures and to make them available to students as podcasts. The advantages are obvious. Students can choose when they wish to listen to them and can pace themselves. We have found that students can vary by a factor of four in the amount of time they spend listening to the same lecture. On the other hand concern has been expressed that if podcasts are available, students may not attend the live lecture and miss the level of engagement and connection with the teacher that can be a feature of it. Recordings of lectures might be better replaced by a carefully designed instructional programme developed to meet a student's needs but this is more difficult and expensive to prepare.

In the case of the live lecture another issue that has been debated is whether students should be allowed to engage with their computers and with electronic devices during the lecture. While such devices may be used to enrich the experience, the student may be distracted by texting, emails and playing video games. On both this issue and the recording of lectures opinion is divided.

The 'flipped classroom'

What is a 'flipped classroom'?

A significant development in recent years has been the concept of a 'flipped classroom' (Figure 23.2). Scarcely a conference on medical education goes past without this being on the agenda. The term was first used in 2007 by chemistry teachers Jonathan Bergmann and Aaron Sams. They argued that students need to have their teachers present so that they can answer questions or provide help if there are aspects of a topic where a difficulty arises. However, students do not need their teachers present in order to listen to a lecture or to review content. They proposed that in the 'flipped classroom' students watch recorded lectures for homework and then engage in further work and discussions in class with their teacher.

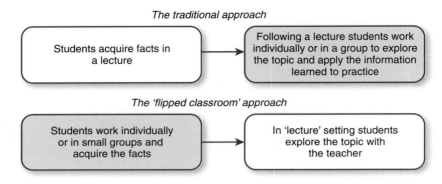

The traditional approach

Students acquire facts in a lecture → Following a lecture students work individually or in a group to explore the topic and apply the information learned to practice

The 'flipped classroom' approach

Students work individually or in small groups and acquire the facts → In 'lecture' setting students explore the topic with the teacher

Figure 23.2 A comparison of the traditional lecture and the 'flipped classroom'

In *Best Practices for Teaching with Emerging Technologies*, Pacansky-Brock (2013) described the concept:

> 'The flipped classroom model uses video recordings of lectures that are shared with students before class time, freeing up face-to-face time to interact with students and apply the information learned in the videos. Ultimately, class-room time is transformed from a passive to an active experience and the role of the instructor shifts from "sage on the stage" to "guide on the side".' (2013: p2)

Application in medical education

Experience has shown that the flipped classroom approach can be applied to medicine and may even be a building block for curricular reform (Hurtubise et al. 2015).

Advantages and disadvantages of the flipped classroom

The advantages of the flipped classroom outweigh the disadvantages. *The advantages* include:

- Students take ownership of their learning.
- Learning is personalised to the needs of the individual student. Students can work at a pace and place to suit them according to their preferred learning style.
- Learning takes centre stage and students get multiple opportunities in the large group sessions that follow the preparatory work to demonstrate their understanding of the topic.
- A focus is an understanding of a topic and in the application of the principles to practical examples rather than simply an acquisition of information.
- Students receive important feedback and areas of difficulty can be identified with remediation provided as necessary.
- The approach provides teachers with the opportunity to engage with students and to get a greater buzz from their face-to-face teaching.

The disadvantages include:

- Students must be disciplined to study the topic using the resources recommended prior to attending the whole class sessions.
- The preparation of the learning resource material to an acceptable standard takes time and some teachers may be concerned about criticisms from their peers when the material is made available.
- The programme for the whole-class session requires careful planning and the teacher may feel uncomfortable with the level of uncertainty.

Implementation in practice

It has been demonstrated that a major curriculum reform is not necessary to implement a flipped classroom. A teacher can implement a flipped classroom for one or more of their lectures.

Careful thought and planning is necessary if the flipped classroom is to be a success:

- Time should be scheduled for students to study the resource materials prior to the large group session.
- The learning outcomes should be made explicit.
- Ideally a choice of resources should be available to students. This could include recordings of the lecture, learning resources prepared for the purpose and online texts.
- Before the classroom session, students can engage by writing notes, identifying a question or issue for consideration by the class later and discussing the topic with their peers.
- Options during the classroom sessions include consideration of questions or issues raised by students, consideration of areas of difficulty, a review of learning outcomes, an in-depth discussion of selected topics or key issues and application of the knowledge gained to new problems.

Over to you

Reflect and react

1. How would you rate your ability as a lecturer? What might you do to improve your performance?
2. Have you evaluated your performance from the perspective of your students or your peers?
3. What do you see as the main purpose of your lecture – to inform the students, to encourage them to reflect and think or to influence their attitudes to the subject?
4. Have you considered adopting a 'flipped classroom' approach for one or more of your lectures? How does this approach meet the FAIR principles for effective learning described in Chapter 3?

Explore further

Journal articles

Harden, R.M., 2008. Death by PowerPoint – the need for a 'fidget index'. Med. Teach. 30, 833–835.

Some practical hints on the use of PowerPoint in presentations.

Hurtubise, L., Hall, E., Sheridan, L., et al., 2015. The flipped classroom in medical education: engaging students to build competency. J. Med. Educ. Curr. Dev. 2, 35–43.

Malik, A.S., Malik, R.H., 2012. Twelve tips for effective lecturing in a PBL curriculum. Med. Teach. 34, 198–204.

Moffett, J., 2015. Twelve tips for 'flipping' the classroom. Med. Teach. 37, 331–336.

Nielsen, K.L., Hansen, G., Stav, J.B., 2012. Teaching with student response systems (SRS): teacher-centric aspects that can negatively affect students' experience of using SRS. Res. Learn. Tech. 21, 211–223.

Recommendations on the use of response systems in lectures.

Owston, R., Lupshenyk, D., Wideman, H., 2011. Lecture capture in large undergraduate classes: student perceptions and academic performance. Internet High. Educ. 14, 262–268.

The advantages and disadvantages of recording lectures.

Robertson, L.J., 2000. Twelve tips for using a computerised interactive audience response system. Med. Teach. 22, 237–239.

Sharma, N., Lau, C.S., Doherty, I., et al., 2015. How we flipped the medical classroom. Med. Teach. 37, 327–330.

Vincent Lau, K.H., Fallar, R., Friedman, E., 2015. Characterizing the effective modern medical school lecture. Med. Sci. Educ. 25, 107–112.

A study of lecture characteristics that correlate best with student satisfaction.

Guides

Brown, G., Manogue, M., 2001. Refreshing lecturing: a guide for lecturers. AMEE Medical Education Guide No. 22. Med. Teach. 23, 231–244.

Nelson, C., Hartling, L., Campbell, S., et al., 2012. The effects of audience response systems on learning outcomes in health professions education. A BEME systematic review: BEME Guide No. 21. Med. Teach. 34, e386–e405.

Books

Bergmann, J., Sams, A., 2012. Flip Your Classroom. ISTE, Arlington, VA.

The seminal text on the flipped classroom.

Bligh, D.A., 2000. What's the Use of Lectures? Jossey–Bass, San Francisco.

A classic text on the use of lectures.

Pacansky-Brock, M., 2013. Best Practices for Teaching with Emerging Technologies. Routledge, New York.

The advantages of small group teaching outweigh the problems that can arise. Conducted appropriately, small group sessions can be successful, but be aware that the teacher's role should be one of facilitator.

What is small group teaching

Small group teaching has been a feature of education programmes for many years, particularly in the clinical context. With the introduction of problem-based learning (PBL) and team-based learning (TBL), small group teaching attracted renewed interest. Learners work together in a group, interacting to achieve common learning goals. A tutor may facilitate the work of a group or the group may be self-directed.

Role of small group teaching

Small group teaching should be included in the teacher's tool kit. Students working in small groups can master learning outcomes not readily achievable using other learning methods. Learning outcomes achieved through small group teaching include:

- The development of social and interpersonal skills and communication skills such as listening and debating. These skills have been recognised as important learning outcomes to be addressed in an educational programme.
- The ability of a student to work as a member of a team and to recognise the roles of other team members. Students are encouraged in small group work to behave in a professional manner and to respect the views of others in the group. Doctors need to work effectively as team members and the skills that enable them to do so should not be taken for granted.
- The ability for students to engage in problem solving, critical thinking, the analysis of a complex issue and refining their understanding.
- The fostering of skills required by students to cope with uncertainty. This reflects medical practice, where issues are frequently complex and uncertainty not uncommon.
- Innovative thinking, creativity and the development of new ideas.

- Deep learning with a more complete understanding of the subject rather than superficial learning where there is an emphasis on memorisation.
- Students reflecting on their own abilities and attitudes and exploring further the concept of professionalism in medical practice. Members of the group may find preconceived beliefs challenged.
- Students' ability to take responsibility for their own learning.

Advantages of small group teaching

Small group work offers a number of advantages:

- Small group learning addresses learning outcomes as described above, that are less easily met by other teaching methods.
- Small group learning embraces the FAIR principles of effective learning as described in Chapter 3. In particular it encourages active rather than passive learning and provides learners with immediate feedback with regard to their understanding of a subject.
- Students find working in properly organised small groups engaging and motivating and are encouraged to continue further with their learning. The approach does place demands on the students but they find the less formal atmosphere of group work more relaxed and conducive to learning. The experience may even be enjoyable.

Small group work draws and builds on the expertise and talents of the members of the group. The less effective and efficient learners may learn from others in the group and improve their learning skills. Studies have shown that where a number of groups have addressed a problem, the results from the 'poorest' group are invariably better than the results from the best individual student working alone.

Problems with small group teaching

Working with small groups can be problematic. Teachers may not use the method effectively and group sessions may be mismanaged:

- Teachers accustomed to lecturing may be less experienced in the role of facilitator in the small group setting. As a result, small group work deteriorates into mini-lectures.
- Small group teaching is considerably more difficult to manage than a lecture as more attention needs to be paid to individual students' behaviour, personalities and difficulties. Diversity in a group promotes varied and interesting opinions, but it also has the potential to create conflict and may interfere with the proper functioning of the group.
- Scheduling the necessary number of rooms for small group teaching may present a logistical problem. If a class of 180 students has small group activities scheduled at the same time with nine students in a group, twenty small group rooms need to be made available. This is not a problem in

team-based learning as the small group activities take place in a lecture theatre or large demonstration room.

- Excessive demands may be placed on teachers' time requiring a higher than normal teacher–student ratio. This can be less of a problem if there is greater emphasis placed on student-directed groups, or if one teacher, as in the team-based learning approach, manages a number of small groups.
- Students too often are not briefed before a small group session about the benefits to be gained and the expected learning outcomes. As a result they may not value what they learn in the small group work and may consider it to be a less effective use of their time compared with attending a lecture or reading a textbook.

Techniques used in small group work

A number of approaches can be used to organise a small group session. Some will be more applicable than others, depending on the situation, the learners, the local context and the expected learning outcomes:

- **Brainstorming**. This is a creative thinking exercise in which group members generate as many ideas as possible without criticising or questioning their validity until time or ideas are exhausted. The ideas are then discussed. This approach is especially valuable to encourage creativity and generate new ideas.
- **Snowballing**. Learners work initially in pairs to discuss the issue or task. They then join with another pair to compare and contrast their results. The group of four learners then combine with another group of four and the exercise is repeated. The deliberations are finally discussed in a plenary session. Snowballing particularly encourages clarification of ideas and values in a non-threatening situation. A variation of snowballing is the jigsaw group. With this technique, after a topic is discussed, the groups reform into new groups, with each new group containing one member of the old group.
- **Role-playing**. Students enact a scenario assuming in turn the role of the doctor, nurse or patient. Role-playing is particularly valuable in exploring communication issues and attitudes. The sessions may be videoed and this can be helpful to students who can view and analyse their own performance and learn from it.
- **Journal club**. This approach is frequently used in postgraduate education. Participants are asked to present and comment on recent papers in the medical literature. The group then discuss the comments.
- **Tutorial/seminar**. Tutorials are particularly helpful to enable students to critically probe subject matter in more detail. This helps them to clarify and expand on their understanding. Triggers such as clinical photographs, a video clip or a short student presentation may be used as a springboard for the tutorial. In a tutorial, the group can discuss material that has been covered in a lecture or in a directed self-learning exercise. The tutorial may be focused on aspects of the subject where students have encountered difficulties.

- **Problem-based learning**. Small group work plays a key role in PBL as discussed in Chapter 16. Group discussions are directed around a problem presented to the group. The students' learning needs relating to the problem are identified.
- **Clinical teaching**. Teaching is conducted with a small number of students around patients in the ward or outpatient department. Clinical skills centres also provide the setting for clinical teaching, with small groups using simulated patients and models. Clinical teaching is discussed in more detail in Chapter 26.
- **Team-based learning.** This is described later in the chapter.

Implementing small group work

Facilitating a small group is one of the most skilled tasks the teacher can undertake. The teacher has to guide the work of the group without dominating it and encourage the learners to interact.

There has been much discussion, particularly in the context of PBL, on whether the group facilitator should be a content expert or a person who has the facilitating skills without necessarily having content expertise. In most situations content expertise is seen as an important prerequisite for the teacher. In small group work content expertise on its own is insufficient. It is important that a teacher has an understanding of the small group process and the necessary facilitation skills.

Some teachers are better than others at running small group sessions and some medical schools or postgraduate institutions prefer to use as group facilitators only teachers who excel in this area. There should, however, be a staff development programme in place to help teachers acquire the skills involved.

Listed below are the tasks that should be undertaken before, during and after a small group session if it is to be successful.

Before a small group activity

A small group activity may appear relatively informal but to be effective it has to be well planned. The teacher needs to:

- Decide which approach to adopt and what type of activities to include. For example, will there be an element of brainstorming or snowballing?
- Determine the composition and the number of students in the group. Group size can vary but a generally accepted optimum number of students is seven or eight. In some situations this has to be expanded but should probably not exceed twelve.
- Arrange the venue for the group meeting and the seating arrangements that will encourage discussion. Figure 24.1 shows three scenarios. The first is the preferred option and maximises the interaction of the group. The second

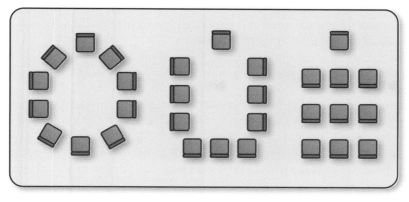

Figure 24.1   Seating plans for small group teaching

emphasises the role of the teacher or group leader. The third replicates a lecture theatre setting and should be avoided.

- Create the right learning environment. For example, noise from adjacent rooms can be a disaster.
- Specify the expected learning outcomes for the session. These will reflect both the subject matter or theme for the group session and also more generic competencies such as reflection and interpersonal skills.
- Ensure that you are familiar with how the small group session relates to the other learning opportunities available to the students.
- Plan the necessary resources, e.g. trigger material in the form of a short video clip, case study or published paper. The trigger may involve real or simulated patients.
- Brief the students in advance if you expect them to do some preparatory work or gain practical experience in the area prior to the small group session.

During a small group activity

There is no one best way of managing a small group and dealing with any problems as they arise. The following guidelines may be helpful:

- The group members should introduce themselves to each other (if the group has not met previously) and state their personal goals and expectations. This sets the scene for the work to be done and can serve as an ice-breaker.
- Review the expected learning outcomes and how these will be achieved. Students may enter the small group activity with some reluctance, feeling the time spent is wasteful and that they will learn better in some other way. One of the common reasons for groups failing is the lack of clear goals and outcomes.
- Establish the ground rules for working as a group, recognising that some people may feel threatened in the group situation. Rules should ensure that contributions are received positively. Typical rules might be that only one member talks at any one time and that all members contribute.

- Create a positive atmosphere for the students' learning. There has to be an atmosphere of mutual trust and respect and students should feel comfortable enough to expose their areas of weakness.
- Focus the group on the task in hand. How this is done will depend on the agreed learning outcomes and group methods adopted. Keep the learning process moving.
- Encourage participation from members of the group by using open-ended questions, listening to what is being said and responding. Monitor the progress of each student in the group.
- Avoid being the centre or focus of the small group activity and do not provide information that other members of the group can provide or that they can get elsewhere.
- Keep the discussion at the appropriate level. It should not be boring or over-challenging.
- Recognise the different roles group members play, for example information provider or influencer, and use this information to help the group accomplish the task.
- Tackle problems in the group, such as a dominant, garrulous or lazy learner, by calling 'time out' and asking the group how they want to solve the issue.
- Towards the end of the session summarise what has been achieved and plan what is expected of the group before they next meet.

After the small group activity

After a small group session teachers need to:

- Support any follow-up actions identified at the group meeting. These may include access to further learning opportunities or communication online between group members.
- Plan any further small group sessions if required.
- Complete any student attendance sheets or student evaluation required.
- Evaluate the small group session, for example through student feedback forms. Reflect on the experience gained by the students and yourself, and consider how the small group session might be improved if it has to be repeated.

Team-based learning (TBL)

What is TBL?

Team-based learning is an approach to small group work that has been adopted in a number of medical schools and has been shown to provide a positive learning experience for students. 'Team-Based Learning is an active learning and small group instructional strategy that provides students with opportunities to apply conceptual knowledge through a sequence of activities that includes individual work, teamwork and immediate feedback' (Parmelee et al. 2012).

TBL can be used with large groups of students divided into multiple small groups directed by one teacher.

Implementation of TBL

TBL involves the following stages:

1. Students' preparatory work prior to the session includes readings, videos, lectures and other learning activities.
2. At the start of the session students are assessed individually using a set of MCQs – the 'Individual Readiness Assurance Test' (iRAT).
3. The students are divided into teams in the classroom or lecture theatre and, following a discussion, answer the same iRAT questions. They receive immediate feedback on the team answers – the 'Team Readiness Assurance Test' (tRAT).
4. The teacher clarifies the concepts relating to questions where students had difficulties.
5. Students, working in the same team, are presented with a practical scenario or problem to which they have to provide answers. The teams display their answers simultaneously to the whole class and the teacher and justify their responses – Team Application (tAPP).
6. The teacher facilitates discussion about the answers and a team can challenge an answer designated to be 'best' – the appeal.

TBL has been compared to PBL; each approach has strong points. Like PBL, TBL involves learning around professionally relevant problems with students learning in small groups or teams. Feedback is given by students and the teacher (Dolmans et al. 2015). A major difference is that in TBL one teacher is responsible for all of the student groups who work simultaneously in one location. This can be in a lecture theatre or accommodation designed for this purpose. In TBL, unlike PBL, students have a mandatory pre-class assignment.

Over to you

Reflect and react

1. Are you making sufficient use of small group methods in your teaching programme?
2. If you are using or considering using small group teaching, look again at the learning outcomes you expect your students to achieve. How do these compare with the suggested outcomes for small group work described above?
3. Which small group methods would be appropriate in your own context and what is your role in the group?
4. Is team-based learning an approach that merits exploring in your own teaching?

Explore further

Journal articles

Burgess, A.W., McGregor, D.M., Mellis, C.M., 2014. Applying established guidelines to team-based learning programs in medical schools: a systematic review. Acad. Med. 89, 678–688.

Dolmans, D., Michaelsen, L., Van Merrienboer, J., 2015. Should we choose between problem-based learning and team-based learning? No, combine the best of both worlds! Med. Teach. 37, 354–359.

Gullo, C., Ha, T.C., Cook, S., 2015. Twelve tips for facilitating team-based learning. Med. Teach. 37, 819–824.

Haidet, P., Levine, R.E., Parmelee, D.X., et al., 2012. Guidelines for reporting team-based learning activities in the medical and health sciences education literature. Acad. Med. 87, 292–299.

McMullen, I., Cartledge, J., Finch, E., et al., 2014. How we implemented team-based learning for postgraduate doctors. Med. Teach. 36, 191–195.

Miflin, B., 2004. Small groups and problem-based learning: are we singing from the same hymn sheet? Med. Teach. 26, 444–450.

Nyindo, M., Kitau, J., Lisasi, E., et al., 2014. Introduction of team-based learning at Kilimanjaro Christian Medical University College: experience with the ectoparasites module. Med. Teach. 36, 308–313.

Steinert, Y., 1996. Twelve tips for effective small-group teaching in the health professions. Med. Teach. 18, 203–207.

Warrier, K.S., Schiller, J.H., Frei, N.R., et al., 2013. Long-term gain after team-based learning experience in a pediatric clerkship. Teach. Learn. Med. 25, 300–305.

Guides

Edmunds, S., Brown, G., 2010. Effective Small Group Learning. AMEE Guide No. 48. AMEE, Dundee.

Parmelee, D., Michaelsen, L.K., Cook, S., et al., 2012. Team-based learning: a practical guide. AMEE Guide No. 65. Med. Teach. 34 (5), e275–e287.

Independent learning 25

Students and trainees should be given more responsibility for their own learning. The learner may require support and direction.

In Chapters 23 and 24 we looked at how students learn in the lecture and small group settings. Here we look at the importance of independent learning where students take charge of their learning and tailor it to their own particular needs. This approach has an important part to play in medical education and should be integrated into the education programme.

The importance of independent learning

There are a variety of reasons for the increased interest in independent learning:

- There has been a move from teacher-centred learning, where the emphasis is on what the teacher teaches, to student-centred learning with the emphasis on what the student learns and where they take more responsibility for their own learning.
- The greater use of strategies such as team-based learning, electives and problem-based learning draws attention to the importance of independent learning.
- The excessive use of lectures as a learning experience has been criticised and there is now more awareness of alternative learning strategies such as the 'flipped classroom' that can be used.
- The move to an outcome-based model, as described in Section 2, has made it easier for students to understand what is expected of them and makes it possible for them to create their own personal learning programme. When asked about the necessity of attending lectures students indicate that the main reason is to learn what they should be studying. In outcome-based education the learning outcomes are transparent.
- There is an increasing focus on distance learning and hybrid models that incorporate face-to-face and distance learning. Independent learning by the student is a key feature.

- Students now learn outside of the medical school including in the community, the district hospital and clinical skills centres. As a result they have to take more responsibility for their own learning.
- With a more diverse student population now admitted to medical school, the learning can be matched to the needs of the individual student.
- The need for lifelong learning and continuing professional development is recognised. From day one of their training, students have to learn to take more responsibility for their own learning and acquire the necessary learning skills.
- Advances in technology and Internet developments have resulted in rich and powerful learning experiences becoming available.

Benefits for the student

Students can benefit in a number of ways:

- They can choose to work at their own pace, spending whatever time is necessary to achieve the required mastery of the subject.
- They can decide when and where they study. This may be in the workplace or at home.
- They can tailor the content of the learning to their personal learning needs.
- They can select the method of learning and an instructional design that best suits them. Some students are visual learners while others prefer the audio channel.
- They can engage to a greater extent in deep learning and reflect on the subject as they pursue their studies.
- They can monitor their own progress, using appropriate learning resources, and adjust their continuing learning based on feedback received.

Independent learning in the curriculum

How much time should be allocated in the curriculum for independent learning? How should independent learning be scheduled? What is the role of the teacher? To what should students be directed or guided? These are questions that need answers.

Time allocated for independent learning and scheduling in the curriculum

Some curricula have formal activities timetabled from 9.00am until 5.00pm, leaving the student free for independent study only outside these times. This schedule is built on the premise that if time is left for private study students will not make full use of it and teachers will be underemployed. Other curricula allow 30% or more of the time available in the curriculum for independent study.

Independent learning can be included in the curriculum:

- As a *replacement for activities such as lectures.* It may be used as a substitute for lectures when a new course is planned or to replace lectures in an existing course to allow students time for other activities.

- As an *alternative option to students' attendance at a lecture.* Podcasts are available for this purpose in many medical schools. Students have the choice of attending the lecture or covering the topic at a time and place more convenient to them.
- As an *adjunct to an existing learning opportunity.* The modern equivalent of the reading list includes URLs for online resources and other multimedia. The teacher can provide annotations and comments to assist the student to select the most appropriate resources.
- For *revision or remedial purposes.*

Directed self-learning and the role of the teacher

The teacher's role in independent learning differs from traditional teaching. There is a switch in emphasis from the teacher as the information provider to the teacher as the facilitator of the students' learning. This role of facilitator is more demanding. The teacher needs to be familiar with the needs of the learners and the potential problems they may encounter when working independently.

Consideration should be given and decisions made whether students have control of their study time or to what extent it should be managed by the teacher. It is important to recognise that although there is no direct teacher contact in independent learning this does not mean that students work without support or in isolation. There are strong arguments for replacing the term 'self-directed learning' with the term 'directed self-learning', as all students benefit from some direction or management of their learning. The need for this will vary from student to student, and with the same student in the different phases of undergraduate and postgraduate education. It has been suggested that the level of autonomy given to a student is one of the most important decisions a teacher has to make. Too little direction will result in confusion and inefficient and ineffective learning. Excessive direction will be demotivating and even result in boredom.

Study guides

The concept of study guides, in print or electronic format, to support a student's learning was introduced in Chapter 15. They can play an important part in independent learning. The design and content of a study guide varies depending on its use. In Figure 25.1 the position on the triangle indicates the extent to which the guide has been designed to:

- help students manage their learning and make the best use of the time available
- suggest activities to facilitate the learning
- provide content to support the students' learning.

The study guide may help students develop the necessary study skills to gain maximum benefit from independent learning.

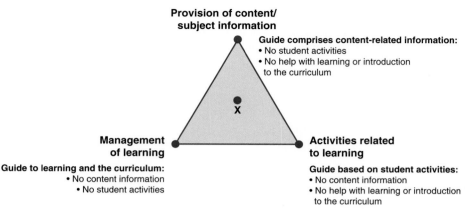

Figure 25.1 The study guide triangle with the three extremes identified and a guide with an equal emphasis on content provision, management of learning and activities represented at X

Learning resources

A wide range of learning resources are available to support independent learning. These include:

- online resources – an increasing amount of learning material is available for instant access through a range of websites, including YouTube, Wikipedia and Facebook; there may be a problem, however, with quality assurance
- recordings and podcasts of lectures
- DVDs – these offer multimedia images including video clips of procedures or personal commentaries from the author
- books and journal articles – print has the advantage that it does not require technology, it is highly portable, and the text can be easily annotated or highlighted
- the curriculum map
- models and simulators
- patients – real, simulated and virtual patients.

The choice of learning resources will depend on the expected learning outcomes, the resources available and the technology support.

Teachers may wish to create independent learning resources for use by their students. It can be a demanding task and is best undertaken in collaboration with an educational technologist or a colleague who has experience in the technology and in instructional design. Just providing students with recordings of teaching sessions is not a satisfactory option. The same general educational principles apply that were described in Chapter 3. Feedback should be provided, learning should be active rather than passive, and the students encouraged to reflect on what they have learned. Students should be able to individualise the resources to meet their own personal needs and the content should be relevant and matched to the specified learning outcomes.

Over to you

Reflect and react

Independent learning has to be carefully planned and not left to chance. This is a significant responsibility for the teacher.

1. Consider whether you have the right balance in your teaching programme between face-to-face contact with your students and opportunities for students to work on their own. Is time scheduled in the curriculum for independent learning?
2. Do you do enough to help the students maximise the benefits of learning on their own through the provision of advice and/or study guides to support the students' learning?
3. Are the benefits to be gained from the use of the new technologies sufficiently exploited in your programme?
4. Consider the level of autonomy that you offer students and the control that you exert over their learning. How does this change as the student progresses through the course?
5. Consider whether you might work on the creation of learning resource material and if so with whom you might collaborate.

Explore further

Journal articles

Al-Hazimi, A., 2012. Development and evaluation of study guide template for an integrated cardiovascular module. Med. Teach. 34 (S1), S6–S13.
A well-designed study guide may be effective as a student learning tool.

Khamseh, M.E., Aghili, R., Emami, Z., et al., 2012. Study guides improves [sic] self-learning skills in clinical endocrinology. Med. Teach. 34, 337–338.

Montemayor, L.L.E., 2002. Twelve tips for the development of electronic study guides. Med. Teach. 24, 473–478.

Guides

Harden, R.M., Laidlaw, J.M., Hesketh, E.A., 1999. Study guides: their use and preparation. AMEE Guide No. 16. Med. Teach. 21, 248–265.

Books

Dron, J., 2007. Control and Constraint in e-Learning: Choosing When to Choose. IDEA Group Publishing, London.
A useful discussion of how much autonomy should be given by the teacher to students to manage their learning.

Websites

Thomas, L., Jones, R., Ottaway, J., 2015. Effective practice in the design of directed independent learning opportunities. Higher Education Academy. <https://www.heacademy.ac.uk/node/10750>.
Research shows benefits of independent learning.

*Lack of planning coupled with poor supervision and feedback
often blights clinical teaching.*

Changing perceptions of clinical teaching

Clinical teaching focuses on real patients in clinical settings. The setting may be
the hospital ward, outpatient department, surgical theatre or the community. Students enter medicine to become doctors, and learning with patients and from
patients is a powerful and effective learning experience. It emphasises a holistic
approach to medical care, requiring from the student the necessary knowledge, skills
and attitudes. Clinical teaching should be at the heart of medical education but how
it is delivered is sadly often ignored.

In earlier chapters we have looked at the apprenticeship model, at the need for a
more authentic curriculum based around patients, at interprofessional learning
opportunities and at the longitudinal clinical clerkships where students have continuity of learning over a period of up to a year in one clinical attachment.

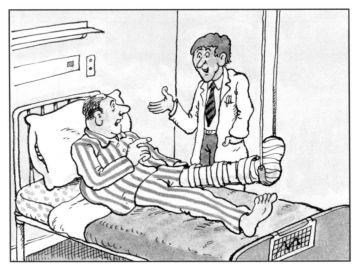

Figure 26.1 Clinical teaching

In postgraduate education there is now recognition that the education of the trainee need not conflict with his or her service role in the delivery of health care. With an appropriate curriculum and planning, learning can be managed 'on the job' in the context of the trainee's work.

The key players in clinical teaching are the student, the teacher and the patient. The coming together of a student enthusiastic to learn, a teacher passionate to teach and a patient willing to contribute provides a powerful and rich learning opportunity for the student.

The student

The role of the student in the clinical setting varies depending on their seniority and stage in the curriculum. A junior student may actively engage in learning while not being a member of the team delivering the patient's care. Students may visit the ward in groups of six to ten and be taught on one or more selected patients by an assigned clinical teacher. Students observe the teacher taking a patient's history or examining the patient and may have the opportunity to do so themselves. The students are then questioned on the findings and required to reflect on the patient's case. Feedback is given to the student.

A more senior student participates in a clerkship as a member of the healthcare team. The teaching is integrated into the care of the patient. Students move from a peripheral role to one of participating as members of the medical community or practice. Students learn from working alongside experienced practitioners and other members of the healthcare team. In the process they are socialised into the practice of medicine. The ward round and patient care conferences are typical learning opportunities.

In postgraduate training, work-based learning is the norm, with trainees developing their competencies as junior members of the healthcare team with certain assigned responsibilities. Short training sessions relating to specialised aspects of the work or procedures can be scheduled.

The teacher

The role of the clinical teacher is challenging. The teacher requires:

- expertise in the area of medical practice
- an understanding of how they can facilitate student learning
- an awareness of the local curriculum and expected learning outcomes for the student
- a recognition of their position as a role model for students.

Junior and senior doctors, other healthcare professionals and students can all contribute to the teaching programme. The role of peer or near-peer teaching is described in Chapter 29.

Table 26.1 The attributes of a clinical teacher

Good clinical teacher	Bad clinical teacher
Plans the clinical teaching with clearly defined learning outcomes	Opportunistic and haphazard approach with no clear plan
Appears enthusiastic with a positive attitude	Uninterested and regards the teaching as a chore or intrusion into other commitments
Serves as a positive role model demonstrating good relationships with patients	Serves as a poor role model lacking aspects of professionalism in practice
Helpful and available to students	Intimidating and teaches by humiliation
Encourages students' active participation	Didactic, with students' role passive
Patient-orientated with problem solving	Disease-orientated and factual
Observes students examining patient and provides feedback	Listens to or reads students' reports of examination of patient and provides inadequate feedback
Provides students with opportunity to practise their skills	Does not encourage students to practise their skills
Tailors the teaching to the stage of training of the students and to the needs of the individual students	Does not take into consideration the stage of training of the students or their individual needs

Many studies have explored the attributes of a good clinical teacher and these are summarised in Table 26.1. The skills required of a clinical teacher too often have been taken for granted and it has been assumed that if doctors are good practitioners, they are also good teachers. Unfortunately this is often not the case, resulting in deficiencies and poor practice in clinical teaching. Problems identified include the lack of planning, inappropriate supervision, lack of feedback to the learner, and a failure to appreciate basic education principles and how students learn.

The patient

The patient is a key element in clinical teaching and may be a hospital inpatient, outpatient or may be located in the community. It is important to obtain full patient consent before students interact with patients and it is important that patients' comfort and dignity are respected. In addition to learning with 'real patients', students can benefit from working with simulations, including simulated patients, manikins and computer representations, as described in Chapter 27. These tools can complement but not replace experience with real patients; they bring the real world into teaching, provide more authentic learning experiences and help to ensure that the teaching is relevant. Patients as well as the teacher can provide feedback to the student about their techniques, attitude and communication skills.

The range of patients seen by students in a clinical attachment should reflect the expected learning outcomes. This can be recorded in a portfolio and any gaps identified in a student's clinical experience should be remedied. Students who use an electronic hand-held device to document their patient encounters produce a more complete record. Patients can be selected for clinical teaching on the basis of their presenting problems, their availability and their willingness and ability to cooperate with students. Patients may actually feel they have benefited from the experience.

Teaching procedural skills

Acquiring experience in procedural skills such as intravenous cannulation or stitching a wound is an essential learning outcome. It is important particularly in the context of the increasing emphasis on patient safety.

A six-step framework for procedural training has been proposed (Sawyer et al. 2015):
1. *Learn* –acquire the necessary knowledge
2. *See* – observe the procedure
3. *Practise* – develop the skill on a simulator
4. *Prove* – demonstrate mastery of the skill on a simulator
5. *Do* – perform the procedure on a patient, initially under supervision
6. *Maintain* – continue clinical practice on patients and simulators to ensure there is not degradation of the skill.

Student progression

In the traditional curriculum, clinical teaching took place in the later years following a study of the basic sciences in the earlier years. Now clinical teaching in many medical schools starts from year 1 of the curriculum. Over the course of the curriculum:

- the clinical teaching assumes a more dominant role in the education programme
- the clinical experiences and attachments increase in length from a half day to weeks or months
- students have increasing responsibility for patients and are assigned roles in the workplace; this may be reflected in specified Entrustable Professional Activities (EPAs), as described in Chapter 8.

Planning and implementing

As with all teaching approaches, planning is important.

- The expected learning outcomes must be clearly defined and communicated to the student. These may include skills in history taking, mastery of practical procedures and an understanding of ethical issues.
- Appropriate learning opportunities, both formal and informal, should be scheduled in the learner's work plan.
- Teachers responsible for a formal teaching session should make the necessary arrangements for the session and should arrange for someone to cover their other commitments so that they are not interrupted by bleeps or other calls.

In a formal clinical teaching session students should be actively involved and engaged. They should feel free to ask questions and ask for help if required. They should be encouraged to reflect and think about the patients they see. Students can be helped to do this by the use of skilful questioning by the teacher, the aim of which includes:

- Arousing the learner's interest, e.g. 'How often do you think a general practitioner will see a patient with a thyroid problem?'
- Testing the learner's knowledge of the subject, e.g. 'Is this a reliable indicator that the patient is hyperthyroid?'
- Promoting the student's understanding and encouraging the student to reflect on the topic and stimulate their critical thinking, e.g. 'Which of the treatment options available would you advise in this case and for what reason?'
- Encouraging the learner to relate theory to practice, e.g. 'What is the explanation for the patient's tachycardia?'
- Inviting comparisons or different viewpoints, e.g. 'What is different in this patient from the last patient we saw?'
- Consolidating the learning through encouraging the trainee to review and summarise the learning that has occurred, e.g. 'What have you learned today from the experience?'

As a teacher you need to learn to be comfortable with silence. Give the students at least 3–5 seconds to think between asking a question and expecting an answer. Insufficient attention is paid to the art of questioning in staff development programmes. We have found the skill lacking even in experienced teachers.

As well as questioning the learner, it is important for the teacher to be a good listener. You need to hear and understand what is being said and respond accordingly. Non-verbal behaviours are also important, so try to maintain eye contact with the student.

Feedback is an essential part of the learning process and in clinical teaching the provision of feedback to the learner is of particular importance. It provides students and trainees with information about their performance and how they can improve upon it. It needs to be given skilfully if you want to motivate your students and this is discussed further in Chapter 3.

Clinical supervision

In postgraduate training programmes, the trainee's clinical supervisor provides the trainee with guidance and feedback on matters of personal, professional and educational development in the context of the provision of safe and appropriate patient care. Clinical supervision of the trainee is important, but how it is carried out is highly variable. The clinical supervisor is responsible for:

- finding out the aspirations and career intentions of the trainee
- recognising the strengths and weaknesses of the trainee and adapting the training to the trainee's needs

- meeting regularly with the trainee to discuss the expected learning outcomes
- monitoring the trainee's progress and giving frequent and constructive feedback
- encouraging the trainee to be reflective by keeping a diary or portfolio of the clinical cases encountered
- being available for the trainee when support or advice is required
- offering counselling to the trainee if the need arises
- keeping the trainee motivated by being positive themselves
- keeping their personal knowledge base and practice up to date.

Over to you

Reflect and react

1. Is clinical teaching provided from the first year of your curriculum and in an appropriate form?
2. Think about how you can ensure that your students or trainees achieve the expected learning outcomes when much of their clinical experience is opportunistic.
3. Is sufficient care taken to inform and obtain consent from patients who participate in the clinical teaching and are they asked for feedback?
4. Do you adequately monitor the progress of students or trainees for whom you are responsible and provide them with frequent and constructive feedback?

Explore further

Journal articles

Dolmans, D.H.J.M., Wolfhagen, I.H.A.P., Essed, G.G.M., et al., 2002. The impacts of supervision, patient mix, and numbers of students on the effectiveness of clinical rotations. Acad. Med. 77, 332–335.
The effectiveness of clinical rotations depends on high-quality student supervision.
Irby, D.M., Papadakis, M., 2001. Does good clinical teaching really make a difference? Am. J. Med. 110, 231–232.
Sawyer, T., White, M., Zaveri, P., et al., 2015. Learn, see, practice, prove, do, maintain: an evidence-based pedagogical framework for procedural skill training in medicine. Acad. Med. 90, 1025–1033.
A six-step approach to learning a procedural skill.

Sutkin, G., Wagner, E., Harris, I., et al., 2008. What makes a good clinical teacher in medicine? A review of the literature. Acad. Med. 83, 452–466.

Guides

Dornan, T., Littlewoods, S., Margolis, S.A., et al., 2007. How Can Experience in Clinical and Community Settings Contribute to Early Medical Education? A BEME Systematic Review. BEME Guide No. 6. AMEE, Dundee.
Ramani, S., Leinster, S., 2008. Teaching in the clinical environment. AMEE Guide No. 34. Med. Teach. 30, 347–364.

Simulation of the clinical experience 27

Simulated patients, manikins, models and computer simulations all complement experience with 'real' patients and have a place in a training programme.

A key element in clinical teaching, as highlighted in the previous chapter, is the patient. Simulated patients, patient manikins or models and virtual patients are widely used and have been found to be of value in undergraduate education and postgraduate training to complement the students experiences with real patients. It is essential that teachers are trained in their use to ensure that students gain maximum benefit from them.

In this chapter we look at different types of simulation, the educational strategies that need to be adopted and the concept of the clinical skills centre. We will first look at the reasons for using simulators in your teaching.

Reasons for simulation

Simulation is an essential rather than an optional element in the curriculum:

- 'Real patients' may not always be available for clinical teaching. With changes in healthcare delivery, patients' stays in hospital are now shorter and during their stay they are occupied with investigation and treatment procedures. Patients may be less willing to have repeated exposure to students.
- A simulated experience can be made available to students at the most appropriate time to fit in with their learning programme. This is not something you can do with 'real' patients.
- With simulation every student can receive a guaranteed and standard clinical experience.
- Repetitive practice is recognised as a key element in the acquisition of clinical skills. Learners can practise with the simulator until they have achieved the necessary mastery of the skill.
- Students are now introduced to clinical experiences earlier in many curricula and preparation on simulated patients and simulators has been shown to prepare them for their work with real patients.

- Trainees can be exposed to uncommon situations or rare clinical events that they may not encounter in their routine clinical experience.
- The management of crisis events can be practised and rehearsed so that students and trainees are better prepared should such events occur in real life. Airline pilots are trained in this way and simulators enable the pilots to deal with extreme situations such as engine failures.
- Students can learn a procedure in a risk-free environment. Learners can make mistakes and appreciate their consequences without causing harm to patients. In some areas it is now a requirement that a doctor demonstrates mastery of a procedure on a simulator before being approved to perform it on a patient. Uncoupling injury from learning sends a message to the public that patients are not 'a commodity' for training.
- Doctors need to be able to work as a member of the team. Simulation can address not only the acquisition of individual technical skills but can also be used to train the learner to work in a coordinated and effective manner as a member of the team.
- The assessment of a learner's mastery of a clinical skill is important. Simulated patients and simulators can be used for this purpose in examinations, including high stakes examinations, to assess the learner's mastery of a skill.
- Simulation can be used to provide students with a motivating and engaging learning experience. The experience can be designed to challenge the students, encourage their reflection and provide feedback about their performance. The experience can be customised to meet the needs of the individual learner.

Simulating 'real' patients

You can simulate the real patient by using:

- **Simulated patients.** Individuals are trained to play the role of a patient.
- **Simulators or manikins.** Devices or models represent the functioning of the body or part of the body and the student interacts with the device.
- **Virtual patients.** The patient is represented in a computer simulation.
- **A hybrid approach.** A simulated patient is combined with a simulator, e.g. a catheterisation model. The student catheterises the 'patient', while at the same time communicating about the procedure with the simulated patient (Kneebone, 2002).

Simulated patients

A simulated patient is a person who has undergone various levels of training to portray a role or mimic a particular physical sign for the purposes of teaching or assessment. The term 'standardised patient' has been used when the person has been trained to play the role of a patient consistently and according to specific criteria. This may be important in the context of assessment.

Students interact with simulated patients as though they are taking a history from a real patient or examining or counselling them. Uses of simulated patients include:

- Teaching and assessing history taking and communication skills. This may include counselling a patient in a difficult or sensitive area such as cancer where the use of a real patient would be inappropriate.
- Teaching and assessing skills in physical examination. This may include teaching and assessing intimate examination of the genitalia.

Barrows (1993) and others have described how simulated patients can mimic a wide range of physical findings from an acute abdomen to spasticity. Simulated patients can be trained to portray various levels of difficulty appropriate to the stage of the learner. The simulated patient may provide a simple account of his or her history on being questioned by the learner, or the patient can be programmed to be aggressive and difficult with a confusing or muddled history. Simulated patients can be trained to represent different settings of care, including ambulatory care and general practice. A special group of simulated patients are recruited specifically to provide students with opportunities to learn the skills of male and female genital and digital rectal examination and female breast examination.

Ward simulation experiences with simulated patients and ward staff have been used in Dundee Medical School to determine whether the final year medical students have acquired the level of clinical ability needed to provide high-quality patient care.

A significant advantage of simulated patients is that the patient can be trained to provide students with feedback about their performance.

Recruiting and training simulated patients

Simulated patients may be professionally trained actors, lay volunteers or healthcare professionals. The training of simulated patients takes time and effort and with a new recruit it is estimated that about 2–3 hours is required to deliver a good simulation. More detailed training may be necessary if the simulation is complex or if the simulated patient is required to assess the student's performance and provide feedback. Some Clinical Skills Units develop and maintain a bank of simulated patients.

Real patients may be trained to present their history and findings for the purpose of teaching and assessment in the same way as simulated patients.

Simulators (manikins and models)

Over the last two decades, manikins or models have been increasingly used to simulate 'real' patients in the teaching of clinical and practical skills and are now part of mainstream medical education. Simulators enable learners to practise patient care in a controlled and safe environment. The level of sophistication of the manikins and models varies. At one end of the spectrum are task trainers, which are designed to teach a low complexity procedure or skill such as breast examination, prostate examination, wound closure, catheterisation or injection techniques. At the other end of the spectrum there are sophisticated models such as 'Harvey' – a life-sized

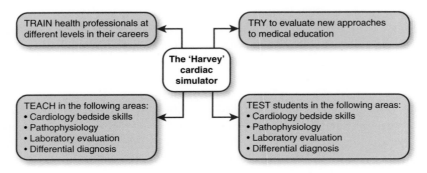

Figure 27.1 Examples of the uses of the 'Harvey' cardiac simulator

cardiovascular patient simulator that can depict the auscultatory, tactile and visual findings for a broad range of cardiac problems (Figure 27.1).

In computer-enhanced manikin simulators computers are integrated into whole- or part-body manikins, controlling the model's physiology and with the output shown as graphic displays on a monitor. A range of clinical scenarios can be set up. A further development is the use of computer-based haptic systems that provide learners with tactile sensations.

Simulators vary in their sophistication with regard to the extent to which they mimic the real-life situation, whether they provide feedback to the learner and the range of tasks and abnormalities that can be simulated. Some skill simulators combine haptics and virtual reality to recreate the clinical environment with visual clues available in real clinical contexts. Work is ongoing to develop virtual reality immersive simulation where the learner is able to interact as if they were in the clinical setting.

There is good evidence that skills gained from practice on a simulator transfer to real patients. Issenberg et al. (2005) in a systematic review of the use of simulators identified key features that contribute to their educational effectiveness:

- **Provision of feedback**. Not surprisingly this was identified as an important feature of simulation-based medical education. (Feedback, the 'F' in 'FAIR' was discussed in Chapter 3).
- **Repetitive practice**. Simulators provide an opportunity for learners to engage in *deliberate practice* where the learner engages in focused and repeated practice with the learning outcomes clearly defined. (Activity, the 'A' in 'FAIR').
- **Individualised learning**. The learning on the simulator should be adapted to individual learning needs. This may mean that some students will require longer time and more practice on the simulator than others. The level of difficulty of the presentation on the simulator may also be altered to match the needs of the student. (Individualisation, the 'I' in 'FAIR').
- **Capture of clinical variations**. A wide variety of problems or conditions can be represented as related to clinical practice. (Relevance, the 'R' in 'FAIR').

- **Curriculum integration**. Simulation-based learning is most effective when it is embedded in the curriculum and not seen as some extraordinary event
- **A non-threatening environment**. The use of simulators is most valuable where mistakes by learners are expected and not criticised, and where these are regarded as 'teachable moments'
- **Defined outcomes**. The expected learning outcomes for using the simulator should be defined and related to the overall outcomes of the curriculum.

Virtual patients

Virtual patients are real patients simulated electronically. They can be used in interactive computer simulations of real-life scenarios. The virtual patient has two components:

- information about the patient, including history, physical findings, laboratory and other investigations and the patient's progress
- the learner's interaction with the case.

With technology developments, virtual patients are now more freely available on the Internet or from commercial sources. In the past the wide range of instructional design and authoring tools had a negative impact on the transferability and sharing of virtual patients between different centres and institutions. Virtual patients developed in one context could not be adapted for use in another context and it was difficult if not impossible for teachers to alter a patient's presentation or investigations to fit in with their own context. There has been a significant move to more collaborative development and sharing of virtual patients with the implementation of a common standards specification. As technology advances it is likely that we will see increasing use made of virtual patients in the training and assessment of students and trainees in all phases of their education.

Uses of virtual patients

Virtual patients can be used in a number of ways, for example:

- to support a traditional curriculum or learning programme, complementing the lecture and clinical experiences
- as the triggers or problem presentation in a problem-based learning curriculum (see Chapter 16)
- to support independent learning, with students individually working through the case scenarios
- in collaborative learning, with students working through a virtual patient scenario in pairs or in a group.

Advantages of using virtual patients

Virtual patients can be accessed on demand, perhaps even more so than simulated patients and manikin simulators, making them a very useful educational tool that offers a number of advantages:

SIMULATION OF THE CLINICAL EXPERIENCE

- Virtual patients can be used to provide students with a wider range of patient scenarios than they may encounter in real life
- The learner can take on the role of the doctor and no harm can result from any mistakes made
- A holistic approach to patient management can be encouraged. The learner can interact with the patient and engage in reflection and clinical reasoning, while at the same time recognising professional and ethical issues
- The virtual patient can highlight the integration of theory and practice, and the basic sciences with clinical medicine
- Virtual patients can be used for teaching and learning and for assessing learners with the learners receiving feedback
- Virtual patients can demonstrate the continuity of care with the same patient located over time in different contexts, including general practice and the hospital setting.

Choice of simulation

A number of factors should be taken into consideration when choosing the simulation approach to be adopted:

- **The expected learning outcomes**. Simulated patients are the obvious choice if communication skills are the expected learning outcome. Computer-based programmes designed for the purpose and virtual patients also have a role to play in communication skills training. If skills in auscultation are the required learning outcome, a manikin such as the Harvey cardiac simulator is appropriate. Virtual patients can contribute to decision making, problem solving and patient management skills.
- **The level of fidelity required**. Simulators vary in how similar they are to the real situation they are designed to simulate. A high-fidelity simulator may be unnecessarily complex and expensive, and a simple piece of plastic simulating a wound on the skin may be adequate to teach suturing skills. A higher-fidelity simulator may be required in a high-stakes examination but may not always be necessary in a training situation. However, students tend to be more engaged with a high-fidelity simulation that more closely resembles a patient.
- **The availability of simulators**. This may be a limiting factor. If students do not have access to a local clinical skills centre with a full range of simulators and a bank of simulated patients, it may be possible to arrange access to a nearby centre. A simulated patient can be trained to meet the needs of a programme but this can be time consuming. Virtual patients that can be shared online across institutions and modified to suit a local context are now available.

Clinical skills centres

There has been a growing interest in the role of clinical skills centres as a setting for teaching and learning clinical skills. These centres are usually a central area housing a range of resources, including simulators and simulated patients that can be used to assist students to master the required clinical skills. The experiences students gain in a centre complement their dealings with real patients in other clinical contexts. Interprofessional education, with joint learning for different healthcare professionals, can successfully take place in the 'neutral setting' of such centres.

Over to you

Reflect and react

1. Simulation is a powerful teaching and learning tool in medical education and a rich variety of simulators are now available. Some of these may be readily available to your students or trainees while others, including high-fidelity manikins, may be available only in a central facility such as a clinical skills unit. What simulators do your students have access to?
2. Could greater use be made in your training programme of simulators, simulated patients or virtual patients? Which of the reasons given for simulation apply in your situation?
3. Are students prepared for their simulated experience in your institution? This includes briefing the students about the expected learning outcomes and what is expected of them in the session. You should familiarise yourself with the simulation prior to the teaching session.
4. Do you debrief the students following the simulation? This is an essential part of the process and will allow you to review what the students have learned and to provide them with feedback.

Explore further

Journal articles

Barrows, H.S., 1993. An overview of the uses of standardized patients for teaching and evaluating clinical skills. Acad. Med. 68, 443–453.

Bath, J., Lawrence, P.F., 2012. Twelve tips for developing and implementing an effective surgical simulation programme. Med. Teach. 34, 192–197.

Berman, N.B., Fall, L.H., Chessman, A.W., et al., 2011. A collaborative model for developing and maintaining virtual patients for medical education. Med. Teach. 33, 319–324.

A description of how virtual patients can be shared between centres.

Huang, G., Reynolds, R., Candler, C., 2007. Virtual patient simulation at U.S. and Canadian medical schools. Acad. Med. 82, 446–451.

Kneebone, R., Kidd, J., Nestel, D., et al., 2002. An innovative model for teaching and learning clinical procedures. Med. Educ. 36 (7), 628–634.

Till, H., Ker, J., Myford, C., et al., 2015. Constructing and evaluating a validity argument for the final-year simulation exercise. Adv. Health Sci. Educ. 20, 1–27.

Ward simulator exercises used at Dundee Medical School.

Guides

Cleland, J.A., Abe, K., Rethans, J.J., 2009. The use of simulated patients in medical education. AMEE Guide No. 42. Med. Teach. 31, 447–486.

Collins, J.P., Harden, R.M., 1998. The use of real patients, simulated patients and simulators in clinical examinations. AMEE Guide No. 13. Med. Teach. 20, 508–521.

Issenberg, S.B., McGaghie, W.C., Petrusa, E.R., et al., 2005. Features and uses of high-fidelity medical simulators that lead to effective learning. BEME Guide No. 4. Med. Teach. 27, 10–28.

Khan, K., Tolhurst-Cleaver, S., White, S., et al., 2011. Simulation in Healthcare Education. Building a Simulation Programme: A Practical Guide. AMEE Guide No. 50. AMEE, Dundee.

Motola, I., Devine, L.A., Chung, H.S., et al., 2013. Simulation in healthcare education: a best evidence practical guide. AMEE Guide No. 82. Med. Teach. 35 (10), e1511–e1530.

E-learning 28

The Internet and resources available online have revolutionised medical education. They can make a significant contribution to your education programme.

A move to e-learning

E-learning refers to 'electronic learning', in which instruction is delivered through a wide range of electronic means, including computer- and Internet-enabled learning. It is now considered mainstream medical education, and is no longer a fad for the technologist or computer enthusiast, or an esoteric application used by a few innovators in the field. It has brought about a paradigm shift in the way our students learn and has become part of and integrated into most educational programmes.

E-learning has been shown to be capable of making a difference with regard to students' learning. Almost every student in a medical school and every trainee doctor spends part of his or her day or week online. They search for information on a topic using Google or some other search engine, communicate with a colleague or teacher, or study a unit, module or course developed in their institution or elsewhere. Medical students will soon all have been born in the 21st century and grown up in a world of digital communication – the digital natives. Teachers born in the 20th century are the digital immigrants (Prensky 2006).

E-learning activities

E-learning is recognised as being more than just technology. It has significant implications for education and includes the social dynamics of networking.

The following examples illustrate the wide range of e-learning activities:

- independent learning using prepared learning modules available online
- accessing information and learning resources online, e.g. YouTube or a Google search
- Web-based synchronous presentation by a teacher to a group of students
- students learning together online in real time, facilitated by a tutor
- asynchronous discussion forums or chat rooms and bulletin boards

- social networks such as Facebook or Twitter
- interactive multimedia activities including games and simulations online or a DVD
- virtual patients with whom the learner has to interact
- videos or audio recordings of lectures distributed through online streaming and podcasts using mobile devices such as smartphones.

Reasons for adopting e-learning

E-learning encompasses a pedagogical approach that can serve as a response to the many challenges and developments confronting medical education. These include:

- the emphasis on student-centred and individualised learning, with 'just-for-you' learning, 'just-in-time' learning and 'just-the-right-place' learning
- the need for distributed learning, with students learning at different sites
- access to medical studies by students from different backgrounds, with programmes required to cater for an increasingly diverse group of students
- international dimensions and globalisation, with an expansion of the traditional classroom to include students from around the world
- advances in medicine with the problem of information overload and the changing emphasis from knowing a fact to knowing where to find it
- acquisition of the skills and tools that learners need to develop in order to prosper in an information society
- the continuum of education from undergraduate through postgraduate to continuing medical education and the need for lifelong learning
- the changing roles of a doctor during their career, with the need to learn new skills and acquire new competencies
- high expectations of students – the 'digital natives' – who come to medical school with more than 10,000 hours' experience in e-learning
- collaborative or peer-to-peer learning, which can be significantly facilitated by social media networking
- interprofessional education with non-threatening learning opportunities online where doctors, nurses and other members of the healthcare team can participate
- sharing of learning resources with potential financial benefits.

E-learning has an important contribution to make in all of these areas and can serve as the solution or be part of the solution to the challenges.

Educational features

E-learning can be designed to deliver more effectively and efficiently what can be learned using more traditional approaches. Alternatively, e-learning can help to bring about a paradigm shift in medical education and serve as a powerful response to the challenges described above. It has been suggested that, like a Trojan horse, e-learning can be introduced not just for the attributes it brings with it but also for the hidden curricular changes included.

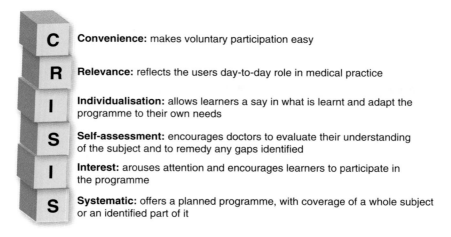

Convenience: makes voluntary participation easy

Relevance: reflects the users day-to-day role in medical practice

Individualisation: allows learners a say in what is learnt and adapt the programme to their own needs

Self-assessment: encourages doctors to evaluate their understanding of the subject and to remedy any gaps identified

Interest: arouses attention and encourages learners to participate in the programme

Systematic: offers a planned programme, with coverage of a whole subject or an identified part of it

Figure 28.1 The CRISIS framework for effective learning

E-learning meets the criteria specified in the CRISIS framework for effective continuing education (Figure 28.1):

- **Convenience**. Students and trainees can learn anytime and anywhere.
- **Relevance**. Theory can be related to practice with on-the-job 'just-in-time' learning. The use of virtual patients extends the learner's clinical experience.
- **Individualisation**. E-learning can be redesigned to meet the needs of individual students in terms of their current requirements, their past experiences and their learning styles.
- **Self-assessment**. Students can be assisted to assess their own competence through questions and assessment opportunities incorporated into the e-learning activity.
- **Interest**. E-learning can be dynamic, engaging and user-friendly if properly developed.
- **Systematic**. An e-learning programme can systematically cover a topic and a curriculum map can be embodied that provides a framework for the student's learning.

Distributed and distance learning

Students may be based at different sites for much of their training programme. This is particularly so in clinical clerkships. Some schools have branch campuses. The availability of school e-learning resources can help to standardise the student's education experience at their different locations and make available learning resources that they could not otherwise access.

Some institutions have put complete courses or modules online. A student may be able to complete a course of study almost entirely at a distance from the course provider. Students working independently have a choice of when and where they study (Figure 28.2). This may be at a central learning resource centre on campus,

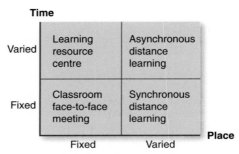

Figure 28.2 In distance learning the place and time of learning may be fixed or varied

in a peripheral training facility at a distance from the teacher and the main campus, or at home. In synchronous learning the time is fixed and students interact live with other students or with the teacher. A typical example of this is a telephone or Web conference or an online chat room. Working asynchronously, students may choose the time at which they wish to learn and communicate with other students and the teacher.

Massive open online courses (MOOCs) have attracted attention in recent years. They aim to give free access online to courses for a large audience and have been provided by some prestigious universities and commercial enterprises. Some MOOCs are available on medical topics. Two types of MOOCs have been identified. The x-MOOC has well-established methods of online learning with tutorials, activities and self-assessment exercises. The c-MOOC is built on networking and connecting and sharing of information between the course participants. In line with the concept of a 'medical school without boundaries', MOOCs offer the possibility of separating teaching from assessment and accreditation.

The extent to which MOOCs will revolutionise university medical education is controversial. E-learning offers the potential sharing of education expertise and can serve as a tool for collaboration as described in Chapter 6 and facilitate the move to 'a medical school without boundaries'.

Blended learning

There is a growing trend in medicine for a blended learning environment where the best of e-learning is combined with the best of face-to-face instruction. We see a convergence between the two learning environments and this may be the single greatest unrecognised trend in higher education today. The challenge for the teacher or trainer is to plan a curriculum that embraces this approach.

Planning a blended approach may mean reconceptualising the role of lectures and placing a greater emphasis on independent learning. It gives the teacher the opportunity to provide students with learning experiences that might not otherwise be accessible to them and to offer a more student-centred approach to learning. In a problem-based learning discussion group, the problem may be presented to the student as an online simulation. When the need for further information is identified during small group work, students can search for this online.

Some medical schools and some postgraduate bodies have made an organisational commitment to blend face-to-face and computer-based learning while others have ignored the opportunities offered. In one school we visited, e-learning had been rejected by the teachers with no e-learning contribution scheduled in the formal curriculum. We found on talking with the students that they were making their own arrangements and on average were spending 2½ hours a day online networking, emailing, or studying material they had personally found on the Web. E-learning is featuring more prominently in the medical curriculum and should not be ignored by curriculum planners or course designers.

E-learning – the educational strategies

To be effective, e-learning requires high-quality content, a robust technology and an appropriate pedagogy. Key to e-learning is the connections created between people. When e-learning has been adopted in medical education the tendency has been to focus on the new technology rather than on the instructional design and educational strategies. We know, however, from past experience that large investments in technology-based initiatives can have disappointing results. A review of one large funding initiative in the UK concluded that inspirational e-learning only results where there is a synthesis of computing, the subject discipline and educational expertise. The presence of these three elements is essential.

In the development of a blended curriculum with the e-learning and face-to-face learning integrated, careful consideration needs to be given to the educational strategies. They may not seem as 'sexy' as cutting-edge technology but they are key to the success of the educational programme. The educational strategies should include (Figure 28.3):

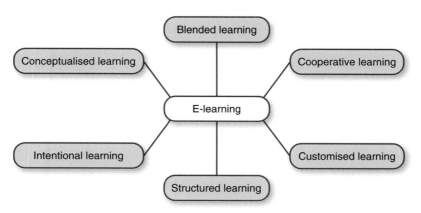

Figure 28.3 Educational strategies and e-learning

- **Intentional learning**. The expected learning outcomes are clearly stated with an explanation of how the learning expected of the student will contribute to achieving their outcomes.
- **Structured learning.** The learning is organised with the relation between the different dimensions specified and an electronic curriculum map used for navigation (see Chapter 22).
- **Contextualised learning**. Theory is related to clinical practice. The curriculum can even be designed around a virtual medical practice with virtual patients (Smith et al. 2009).
- **Customised learning**. Personalised adaptive learning is provided geared to the student's individual needs.
- **Cooperative learning**. Opportunities are scheduled for collaborative learning with students working together locally and internationally.

Over to you

Reflect and react

1. The future is blended learning. As a teacher, think what this means for you in your course and whether you have the optimum face-to-face and e-learning mix.
2. Be aware of the range of tools available, including synchronous and asynchronous online learning, podcasts and social media.
3. Consider your role in e-learning. Do you serve as a role model for your students with regard to accessing information online and using learning resources?
4. Is your aim to make your teaching more effective and efficient using e-learning or is your aim to use e-learning to benefit your students in ways not otherwise possible, for example by personalising their learning? Technology should be a tool to promote learning not an end in itself.

Explore further

Journal articles

Cartwright, C.A., Korsen, N., Urbach, L.E., 2002. Teaching the teachers: helping faculty in a family practice residency improve their informatics skills. Acad. Med. 77, 385–391.

This article describes how teachers can become role models for their students in the area of informatics.

Choo, E.K., Ranney, M.L., Chan, T.M., et al., 2015. Twitter as a tool for communication and knowledge exchange in academic medicine: a guide for skeptics and novices. Med. Teach. 37, 411–416.

A discussion of the potential advantages and the barriers to the use of Twitter in medical education.

Ellaway, R.H., Coral, J., Topps, D., et al., 2015. Exploring digital professionalism. Med. Teach. 37, 844–849.

Ellaway, R.H., Fink, P., Graves, L., et al., 2014. Left to their own devices: medical learners' use of mobile technology. Med. Teach. 36, 130–138.

How learners can use mobile devices across a whole curriculum.

Forgie, S.E., Duff, J.P., Ross, S., 2013. Twelve tips for using Twitter as a learning tool in medical education. Med. Teach. 35, 8–14.

Twitter can be a useful adjunct for more personalised teaching and learning in medical education.

Ilic, D., Bin Nordin, R., Glasziou, P., 2015. A randomised controlled trial of a blended learning education intervention for teaching evidence-based medicine. BMC Med. Educ. 15, 39.

Kind, T., Patel, P.D., Lie, D., et al., 2014. Twelve tips for using social media as a medical educator. Med. Teach. 36, 284–290.

Rasmussen, A., Lewis, M., White, J., 2013. The application of wiki technology in medical education. Med. Teach. 35, 109–114.

Smith, S.R., Cookson, J., McKendree, J., et al., 2009. Patient-centred learning – back to the future. Med. Teach. 29, 33–37.

The use of a virtual practice as a learning tool.

Guides

Ellaway, R., Masters, K., 2008. E-learning in Medical Education. AMEE Guide No. 32. AMEE, Dundee.

E-learning is now part of mainstream medical education.

Books

Clark, R.C., Mayer, R.E., 2007. E-learning and the Science of Instruction – Proven Guidelines for Consumers and Designers of Multimedia Learning, 2nd ed. Jossey–Bass, Chichester.

An introduction to some of the theory underpinning the use of e-learning.

Ellaway, R.H., 2013. Digital medical education. In: Dent, J.A., Harden, R.M. (Eds.), A Practical Guide for Medical Teachers, 4th ed. Elsevier, London. (Chapter 27).

How to best configure medical education in a digital age.

Prensky, M., 2006. Don't Bother Me Mom – I'm Learning! How Computer and Video Games Are Preparing Your Kids for Twenty-first Century Success – and How You Can Help! Paragon House, Minnesota. (Chapter 4).

Sandars, J.E., Frith, G.S., 2013. Mobile learning (m-learning). In: Dent, J.A., Harden, R.M. (Eds.), A Practical Guide for Medical Teachers, 4th ed. Elsevier, London. (Chapter 28).

Exciting new possibilities for teaching and learning on the move.

Reports

Yuan, L., Powell, S., 2013. MOOCs and Open Education: Implications for Higher Education. <http://publications.cetis.ac.uk/2013/667>. JISC CETIS.

This report sets out to help decision makers in higher education institutions gain a better understanding of the phenomenon of massive online open courses (MOOCs).

Peer and collaborative learning 29

Students learning from each other is effective. This can be informal or incorporated into scheduled activities.

Recognition of peer-to-peer (P2P) learning

Watching my 5-year-old grandson learn to use a computer, I (RMH) noted that he did not learn from the instruction manual, from his parents or from instruction at school. He learned from his 7-year-old sister. This is not surprising. Much of what we learn in day-to-day life is from friends and colleagues. It has always been a feature of how students learn at medical school. The difference today is that the value of learning in this way is appreciated and is given a more formal role in the curriculum. Students engaged in peer-to-peer (P2P) and collaborative learning tend to have a greater mastery of the expected learning outcomes with higher test scores, higher self-esteem, greater interpersonal skills and a greater understanding of the content they are studying.

A range of terms such as 'P2P learning', 'collaborative learning' and 'cooperative learning' have been used to describe how students can learn with and from each other in formal and informal settings. Distinctions are sometimes drawn between the terms but frequently they are used interchangeably.

P2P learning

P2P learning has been defined by Topping (1996) as 'people from similar social groupings who are not professional teachers helping each other to learn and learning themselves by teaching'. In near-peer-assisted education programmes, the teacher is a trainee or student one or more years senior to another student. In P2P learning one student assumes the role of teacher or tutor while other students assume the role of learners or tutees. Students may switch their role from tutor to tutee. Usually, to guide students in their role as tutor, some instruction is given in teaching skills.

Collaborative learning

In collaborative learning, students learn from each other without the assignment of specific roles of tutor and tutee. Students work together as members of a group or team to solve a problem, complete a task or create a product. It is through working together that the students learn. There is a sharing of authority and acceptance of responsibility among group members for the group's actions. The group may be assessed by the activity and product of the group rather than the individual's activity or achievements within the group.

The term 'cooperative learning' rather than 'collaborative learning' has been used where there is more structure and organisation given to the group activity but the terms are often used interchangeably.

Examples of P2P and collaborative learning

P2P or collaborative learning may be adopted in the medical curriculum in a range of formats (we have not distinguished between the two approaches as there is often an overlap). Here are some examples:

- Students are given the role of tutor in slots scheduled in the curriculum.
- Students form informal partnerships to assist each other.
- Students work in groups in the context of problem- or team-based learning.
- Students work in pairs facilitating each other's learning.
- Students collaborate in a project or in practical work such as anatomical dissection.
- Students work as members of an interprofessional group in a community-based project.
- Students work online as members of a formal discussion group with a specific task as the focus.
- Students share their experiences and information with others through a social network such as Facebook.
- Students collaborate in the development of educational resources or textbooks that they share with others.
- Students have the responsibility for assessing each other's achievements in an area such as professionalism (peer assessment).
- Students in more senior years or junior doctors teach junior students.

Benefits to be gained by P2P and collaborative learning

The institution or medical school and the learner can benefit in a number of ways if P2P collaborative learning is incorporated in the curriculum:

- Students can learn effectively from their peers, in particular where there are problems relating to handling complex concepts.
- Learning outcomes less easily achieved through other methods are promoted. These include interpersonal skills, communication skills, higher-level thinking skills, skills of critical appraisal and team working skills.
- Students are helped to develop their confidence and self-esteem.

- Students are prepared for lifelong learning as the classroom more closely resembles real-life social and employment situations.
- Students' satisfaction with the learning experience is enhanced, with a more positive attitude developed towards the subject matter.
- Students are encouraged to appreciate diversity and to reflect and appreciate different viewpoints and perspectives brought to the discussion by other students.
- Learners working online at a distance have a supportive community environment.
- Additional support for student learning is provided at a time when there is pressure on staff–student ratios.
- An educational environment is created within the institution where collaboration is valued.
- A student-centred learning approach is supported, with students taking more responsibility for their own learning.
- Teaching is a powerful learning tool – 'to teach is to learn twice'.
- Students feel engaged and have some ownership of the curriculum.
- The concept of the student as an assessor of other students is supported, particularly in areas such as attitudes and professionalism.
- Students receive significant feedback as part of the learning activity, which is not always possible in other situations, particularly in large group learning.
- Students' skills as teachers are developed in line with recommendations from accrediting bodies that medical graduates must be able to demonstrate appropriate teaching skills.
- Experience gained as a student teacher may encourage some students to seek an academic career.

Implementation in practice

The successful implementation of P2P and collaborative learning has much in common with the general curriculum development principles described else-where in this book. It is important to clarify the expected learning outcomes, to ensure that planning and preparation is adequate, that the process is facilitated by an appropriate education environment and that there is a match between assessment, and teaching and learning. Some specific recommendations are noted below.

P2P learning

The following tips contribute to successful P2P learning:

- Incorporate P2P learning formally into the curriculum and do not consider it only as an add-on extra.
- Schedule the P2P sessions and make the necessary arrangements for students to sign up.
- Decide whether students' attendance is obligatory or whether P2P sessions are optional.

- Ensure that both the tutors and tutees are aware of how P2P learning contributes to the mastery of the learning outcomes of the course. It is sometimes claimed that the tutor gains as much if not more than the tutee. This includes mastery of teaching skills.
- Ensure that student tutors are fully briefed and have training in the necessary skills. They may be assisted with the provision of learning resources to support the learning.
- P2P tutors should have ongoing mentoring and coaching by staff.
- Chose the form of P2P learning that is most appropriate for your situation. This may involve students in the same year or more senior students or junior doctors acting as tutors.
- In planning and organising P2P learning, a team approach involving both staff and students is useful.
- As with all learning experiences, P2P should be monitored and evaluated.

Collaborative learning

The success of collaborative learning can depend on how it is implemented:

- Explain to the students the benefits of the collaborative learning approach and the expected learning outcomes, including the development of interpersonal skills and mastery of the subject content. It is important that they accept them.
- Collaborative learning can be at its most effective with heterogeneous groups where students tend to interact and achieve more compared to working with students more closely matched in their abilities and background.
- The learning tasks can be structured so that students must depend on each other for completion of the task. This involves trust building, conflict management, encouragement and negotiation within the group. Each student should be held accountable for doing his or her own share of the work. One interprofessional group we saw, as described in Chapter 18, worked well because the solution to the problem presented required the theoretical knowledge of the medical student members of the group and the practical knowledge of the midwives.
- It is important that sufficient time is allocated to collaborative learning. Students need to complete the required tasks and achieve the expected learning outcomes. This creates an atmosphere of achievement in the group. Some of the social benefits may become apparent only after the group has worked together for a number of weeks.
- Students should have the opportunity within their small group to reflect upon and reply to the diverse responses from other group members. The exchange of views in the group should help students to understand better the issues and concepts being discussed.
- It is important to recognise that just because students are working in small groups it does not mean that they are engaging in collaborative learning. You need to be sure that students are cooperating with regard to their own learning and the learning of others in the group.

- Each member of the group should contribute to the work and product of the group so that the end result will be better than that achieved by one student, even the best, working independently.
- Encourage students in the group to explain the concepts or principles to others and allow for the explanation to be discussed by the group. This can lead to effective learning for the members of the group.
- The group activities should be organised in such a way that the learning success of each individual and the group as a whole is recognised. We saw this achieved in one setting where an individual at the end of the week was chosen by the teacher at random to present the work of the group. The group was given a mark based on the individual's performance. The group had to 'sink or swim' together.
- Monitor the group activity and the progress being made by the students in the group. The teacher, when facilitating a group, should provide assistance and clarification if required. It is important that the teacher does not dominate the session and convert it into a mini-lecture.

Over to you

Reflect and react

1. You may feel uncomfortable delegating teaching responsibilities to a student or trainee. There is overwhelming evidence that this can be effective. Consider how P2P or collaborative learning could be adopted in your situation. Would any of the examples given work?
2. Which of the advantages of P2P or collaborative learning listed apply in your situation?
3. Look at the learning outcomes for your course or curriculum and consider whether some outcomes, such as team work, could be usefully addressed through P2P or collaborative learning.

Explore further

Journal articles

Aba Alkhail, B., 2015. Near-peer-assisted learning (NPAL) in undergraduate medical students and their perception of having medical interns as their near peer teacher. Med. Teach. 37 (S1), S33–S39.
Near-peer-assisted learning has an important role to play.

Klemm, W.R., 1994. Using a formal collaborative learning paradigm for veterinary medical education. J. Vet. Med. Educ. 21, 2–6.
A case study of how small groups of students helped each other to learn.

Stone, R., Cooper, S., Cant, R., 2013. The value of peer learning in undergraduate nursing education: a systematic review. ISRN Nurs. 2013, 930901.
Peer learning was shown to be as effective as the conventional classroom lecture method in teaching undergraduate nursing students.

Topping, K.J., 1996. The effectiveness of peer tutoring in further and higher education: a typology and review of the literature. High. Educ. 32, 321–345.

Turner, S.R., White, J., Poth, C., 2012. Twelve tips for developing a near-peer shadowing program to prepare students for clinical training. Med. Teach. 34, 792–795.

Guides

Ross, M.T., Cameron, H.S., 2007. Peer assisted learning: a planning and implementation framework. AMEE Guide No. 30. Med. Teach. 29, 527–545.

Books

Boud, D., Cohen, R., Sampson, J. (Eds.), 2001. Peer Learning in Higher Education: Learning from and with Each Other. Kogan Page, London.

SECTION 5

Assessment

'Lack of assessment and feedback, based on observation of performance in the workplace, is one of the most serious deficiencies in current medical education practice.'

John Norcini and Vanessa Burch, 2007

- The assessing of the learner is arguably the most important task for the teacher. Students can walk away from bad teaching, but they cannot avoid bad assessment
- An understanding of basic concepts and approaches will help you to do a better job
- Written questions have a role to play alongside other assessment methods
- An assessment of students' clinical competence is key to an assessment of their ability to practise medicine
- Portfolio assessment is a response to changes in medical education including the emphasis on professionalism and the need to give students more responsibility for their own learning
- A range of assessment tools and approaches are available to assist with key selection decisions
- Curriculum evaluation is an essential part of the educational process

An understanding of the basic concepts and approaches to assessment will help you to do a good job.

The importance of assessment

The assessment of a student's or trainee's learning is important for them, for the teacher, the course organiser, the accrediting body and the public. Important decisions are taken about students as a result of the scores they achieve in examinations. Teachers and the other stakeholders need to know if students have achieved the appropriate level of mastery to move on to the next part of their training programme and if, on completion of their training, they are competent to practise as a doctor. Students need to get feedback on their progress.

Assessment is important, but it is one of the most difficult areas in which to get agreement. What constitutes a fair examination and what are the criteria for passing a student? Is the examination assessing what we want to measure? Assessment procedures have been criticised by students, by professional bodies and by those outside medicine. In a recent court case, a judge criticised a nursing school for a failure to identify in its assessment procedures a nurse who proved grossly incompetent and demonstrated unprofessional behaviour after she qualified. For the student, sometimes assessment may be seen as analogous to playing in a cricket match where the rules have not been clearly specified in advance and are constantly being changed by the umpire. Students may perceive meeting the examiner as confrontational and threatening, and view the examiner as someone whose aim is to catch them out and find fault with them.

Where there are problems with assessment, this is serious: students can walk away from bad teaching but they are unable to do so with assessment if they are to achieve the qualification they seek. The fact that assessment is a key and integral part of curriculum development is often not recognised. Assessment should be inextricably linked to the learning outcomes and teaching methods and seen not only as a testing or measurement problem. Course design and assessment are inseparable.

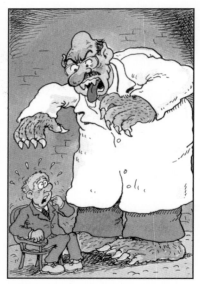

Figure 30.1 Students may perceive the examiner as threatening

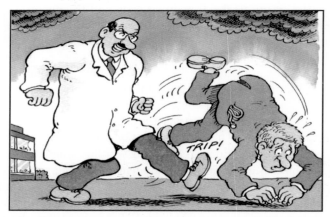

Figure 30.2 Students may perceive the examiner as someone whose aim is to catch them out

When thinking about assessment it is useful to consider six questions. The answers to the questions will determine whether the arrangements made to assess the students' competence meet the standards expected.

1. Why assess the student?
2. Who should assess the student?
3. What should be assessed?
4. How should the student be assessed?
5. When should the student be assessed?
6. Where should the student be assessed?

Why assess the student?

At an early stage in planning an assessment programme it is important to consider the purpose of the assessment. An assessment designed to certify a student's competence to practise as a trainee doctor will be different from the assessment method used to review a student's progress and provide feedback during coursework. Traditionally, assessment has been described as either 'formative', where the main aim is to provide the learners with feedback about their progress, or 'summative', where the aim is to determine whether the learners have achieved the course objectives. This distinction has become blurred with the recognition that summative assessment can also be used to provide feedback to the learner and summative decisions may be based on evidence collected during the training programme.

The purposes that can be served by assessment include:

- **Deciding whether the learner is 'fit for purpose'**. Has the learner satisfactorily completed the training programme and achieved the standard expected by the public and professional bodies to practise as a trainee or as a specialist in a particular field of medicine? Assessment has a key role to play in mastery learning and whether the learner is 'fit-for-purpose'. Basic principles of mastery learning are that the required standards will be achieved by all learners and that little or no variation in measured outcomes will result (McGaghie 2015). This has implications for assessment. In an 'assessment-to-a-standard' or competency-based approach what matters are the standards students achieve rather than the time it takes to do so.
- **Assessing the student's progress during the education or training programme**. A student's deficiencies should be identified early in a training programme so they can be remedied. Waiting until a final examination at the end of training will be too late to take the necessary action. This is particularly true with regard to the assessment of behaviour and attitudes.
- **Grading or ranking the student with the aim of identifying the 'best' students among those being assessed**. This 'norm-referenced' approach to assessment is applicable when candidates have to be selected for a limited number of posts, or students selected for admission to medicine where only a set number of places are available. This approach to assessment should not be confused with a 'criterion-referenced' approach where the learner's achievement is assessed against the expected learning outcomes or a set of criteria and not as a comparison with how other students performed.
- **Enhancing the student's learning**. Assessment can benefit learning in a number of ways. Emphasis is now placed on 'assessment for learning' as well as 'assessment of learning'. In addition to serving as a tool for accountability, assessment can be a tool to support and improve learning. In what is known as 'test-enhanced learning', the act of taking a test and retrieving information from memory can directly increase retention of information. Testing can also help a student to assess what they know and provide feedback for further learning.

- **Motivating the student**. It has been demonstrated that assessment has a powerful impact on students and is a major factor in driving their learning. In Dundee Medical School we found that students paid less attention to the discipline of otolaryngology, because there was no examination on the subject, despite the topic being taught in an imaginative problem-based way. When the subject was routinely included as a station in the final objective structured clinical examination (OSCE), the students' approach to studying the topic changed dramatically.
- **Providing feedback for the teacher**. The teacher can glean useful information from student assessment but all too often this source of information is untapped. The analysis of students' scores in one multiple choice question (MCQ) examination revealed that students had performed badly in a question relating to diabetes. This was subsequently found to be related to a weakness in the training programme, which had to be addressed.
- **Bringing about assessment-led innovation**. Recognising the powerful impact assessment has on the student and the teacher. Changes to assessment can be used to lead changes in the curriculum rather than assessment coming at the end of the curriculum planning process.

Who should assess the student?

One reason why assessment is complex and the teacher's responsibilities may be unclear is that there is a range of stakeholders involved. These include:

- international accrediting bodies
- national accrediting bodies such as the General Medical Council in the UK and the National Board of Medical Examiners in the United States
- professional bodies, for example the Royal Colleges in the UK and the National Boards in the United States
- other healthcare professionals
- the public and patients
- the individual school where the student is enrolled
- the department or course committee responsible for teaching the subject
- the individual teacher
- the students themselves.

In medical schools in the UK, student assessment has been the responsibility of each medical school, with the assessment process overseen by the General Medical Council (GMC). Teachers from other schools serve as external examiners and along with internal examiners participate in the development of the school's examinations, their implementations and pass/fail decisions. In contrast, in North America and in some other countries there is a national examination that students are required to pass. Each approach has merits. A national examination, while setting national standards, may stifle innovation in individual medical schools and there is no evidence that doctors are safer and make fewer errors in countries with a national examination (Harden 2009).

After completing their training, doctors have to take responsibility for assessing their own performance and keeping themselves up to date. Not all doctors have the necessary skills or recognise the importance of this responsibility. Students must be given experience in assessing their own competence as part of their undergraduate education with reinforcement throughout their postgraduate training. Problems with unreliability in self-assessment are well recognised. There may also be problems with how students react to the assessment of their own competence. On one occasion, we asked students to mark their own examination paper against a model answer. Some found the procedure so traumatic that they were unable to complete the process and to our surprise required counselling as a result. Training students to become doctors who are enquirers into their own competence, and who are comfortable with this, should be a required learning outcome of the curriculum.

Increasing attention is being paid to peer assessment. The evaluation of students by their peers against certain learning outcomes has become part of some institutions' assessment strategy. This is particularly valuable in the assessment of attitudes, where often the student body has a better understanding of an individual student's strengths and weaknesses than the teachers.

What should be assessed?

A key feature of outcome-based education, as discussed in Section 2, is that assessment is matched closely with the specified learning outcomes. This should be set out in a blueprint that maps each assessment to the expected learning outcomes.

What we choose to assess in the education programme demonstrates to students what, as teachers, we value. Many problems encountered with assessment arise from a failure to adequately consider what is assessed. Assessment drives learning as we have described above. What is assessed becomes, for students, the course objectives.

In the past the emphasis in assessment was on the knowledge domain with less attention paid to skills and attitudes. There were a number of reasons for this. Mastery of knowledge was traditionally regarded as of greater importance than the development of attitudes. Knowledge was also easier to assess than other domains so there was a natural tendency to assess what was easy and to shy away from areas where assessment was contentious or difficult. Written assessments, including multiple choice question (MCQ) papers that tested the knowledge domain, dominated assessment practice. Someone who can answer correctly a set of MCQs, however, is not necessarily a good doctor. There has been a move to assess the student or doctor's more complex achievements, such as higher-order thinking, clinical skills, attitudes and professionalism.

The introduction of the OSCE stimulated the assessment of psychomotor and other performance-related skills. More recently the adoption of portfolio assessment and multi-source feedback recognised the importance of the assessment of independent learning and self-assessment skills, attitudes and professionalism.

With the many changes advocated in medical education and the different expectations we have of our students in today's curricula, it is important that assessment does not lag behind. What we assess must closely match what we expect students to learn.

Competency-based assessment

The move to outcome- or competency-based education as described in Section 2 necessitates by definition a robust approach to assessment. Doctors will be certified on an assessment of the attained competencies rather than time in training. The assessment tools selected need to be able to assess the student or trainee's mastery of the wide range of specified learning outcomes. In competency-based education, assessment should be embedded in the education or training programme. There should be a greater emphasis on formative assessment, and this should be part of the culture of the programme. Tools will be further developed to better assess on-the-job competencies such as interprofessional and teamwork skills in the context of the complexity of medical practice.

How should the student be assessed?

A wide range of tools or instruments are now available that can be used to assess the student's competence (Figure 30.3). Some of these are described in the chapters that follow. Just as important is the way in which the tool is employed. A good tool badly used will yield inappropriate or misleading results. We now have a better understanding of what makes a good assessment:

- **The method should be reliable and consistent**. This relates to the certainty with which a decision can be made about the student's performance on the basis of the test results. For a reliable assessment the measurement instrument must be relatively stable. It would not be good practice, for

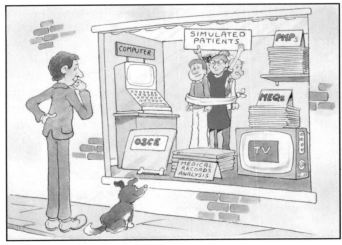

Figure 30.3 A range of assessment tools are available

example, to use an elastic tape measure to measure length. The measurement would not be reliable. High reliability was one of the reasons for the adoption and widespread use of MCQs. Problems with reliability associated with traditional tests of clinical competence were highlighted when we found that examiners watching the same clinical performance awarded different scores to the examinees. Watching a video of the students' performance some weeks later, they were not consistent with the marks they had awarded. The problem of reliability was a factor that stimulated us to develop the OSCE (Harden et al. 2016).

- **The method should be valid.** In other words the assessment method should measure the learning outcomes intended. The test should be an 'honest' one, testing what it purports to measure. An essential element of an 'authentic curriculum', as described in Chapter 12, should be authentic assessment. There may be a trade-off at times between reliability and validity. This is illustrated in the classic story of the drunk man who was seen at night looking under a street light for his car keys which he had dropped. When asked why he was looking there when he had dropped them a short distance away, he replied that it was easier to see what was on the ground under the light. His search strategy, although having some merit, was not valid in his situation. Measurement of an athlete's performance in a high jump is not a valid measure of how the same athlete will perform in a long jump.

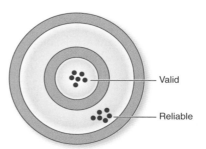

Figure 30.4 Tests should be valid as well as reliable

Unfortunately, in the past reliability has been emphasised at the expense of validity. What is needed is a test that is both valid and reliable. A test may be reliable but it is of no value if it does not measure what we want to measure. Unfortunately, the more simple a test, the more likely it is to be reliable while at the same time the less likely it is to be valid. Medicine by its nature is a complex subject and assessment of professionalism or communication skills is by necessity complex if it is to be valid.

- **The method should be feasible** in terms of the resources available and the number of students to be examined. The assessment scheme should not be overly complex and should be capable of being implemented in routine practice.

- **The assessment should have a positive impact on the student's learning**. When we first introduced the OSCE in the final examination we found that students spent less time in the library revising their theoretical knowledge and more time learning on the wards. This was in line with the aims of the curriculum.

Van der Vleuten and Schuwirth (2005) have described the utility or value of an assessment as a function of these features.

Utility = Reliability × Validity × Feasibility × Education impact × Cost effectiveness

Standard setting

It is helpful to think of assessment in two stages:

- the collection of information about the student's competence, e.g. at stations in an OSCE, in a portfolio or in a written examination, and
- a decision as to whether the student has achieved the standard expected.

There should be a decoupling of the assessment moment and the decision moment.

A standard is a statement of whether a student's examination performance is good enough for a particular purpose. A standard setting strategy should be adopted which serves as a basis for deciding whether a student has reached the standard required to pass the examination. Relative or norm-referenced standards are based on a comparison of a learner's performance with his or her peers: for example, 75% of learners will pass. Absolute standards in contrast are based on the learner's performance in terms of set criteria: for example 60% of the MCQs answered will be correct. Much attention has been focused in recent years on methods of determining the standard expected of students in an examination. Should the pass mark be 60% or should it be 55% or 65% of questions answered correctly? A range of standard setting methods to determine the passing score for an examination has been employed for written and performance tests. These are based on the involvement of and discussions by a group of subject matter experts. Setting pass standards is a complex task and beyond the scope of this book. Useful introductions to setting standards in examinations can be found in the references provided at the end of this chapter.

Programmatic assessment

Given that every individual assessment has severe limitations with regard to the decisions that can be based on the results, van der Vleuten and Schuwirth (2005) proposed that assessment of the student should be undertaken at the level of the programme rather than the individual examination. Information is gathered from individual assessments, seen as individual data points, but decisions are made only when sufficient information from individual data points and assessments is combined. Decisions are made in relation to the expected learning outcomes, e.g.

communication skills or attitudes based on information obtained from multiple sources, including in the case of communication skills an OSCE, Mini-CEX (clinical evaluation exercise) and multiple-source feedback. Information can be collected in a portfolio. Pass–fail decisions are not made on individual data points but these are used to provide the student or trainee with feedback.

When should the student be assessed?

Traditionally learners were assessed on their mastery of the subject in a set examination at the end of the course. Increasing emphasis is now being placed on collecting evidence about the learners' achievement of the expected learning outcomes during their training or course of study. There are a number of reasons for this. Without the time constraints of a final examination, a much wider sample of the students' performance can be assessed, increasing the reliability of the examination. In addition, the assessment may be more valid as the assessment tools that can be adopted during the course may assess the learning outcomes that are difficult to assess in an end-of-course final examination. A key additional benefit of in-course assessment is that it provides feedback to the student and teacher and allows time for remediation.

Less frequently undertaken is the assessment of the student at the beginning of the training programme. A number of years ago we asked third-year students on day one of their course in endocrinology to complete the end-of-course examination. The results were surprising. Some students scored less than 10% while other students scored almost 50%, the pass mark for the examination. This highlighted that courses in endocrinology needed to be tailored to suit the different abilities of the students. Independent learning modules were developed which were used successfully to replace lectures on the topic.

The first occasion we assess students is when we select students to enter medical studies. This is one of the most important assessment decisions and is discussed in Chapter 34.

The progress test

The progress test is an approach to assessment where the student's knowledge is repeatedly assessed at time intervals throughout the course. The features are:

- Questions (either MCQ or constructed response items) assess the knowledge expected of the student on graduation. The test is comprehensive, covering all of the domains of relevant medical knowledge.
- Students from every year in the medical school sit the same examination. The results expected of final-year students are very different from those expected of first-year students.
- Students sit the test at fixed intervals (once or several times per year) and can over time chart their development or progress in different domains.

The progress test was introduced in Maastricht and Kansas City, and is now widely used. The test can provide useful feedback to students and to curriculum evaluators. In Dundee, for example, following the introduction of a new vertically integrated curriculum we were able to show that students' knowledge in relation to the basic sciences increased or remained steady instead of declining.

Progress tests have been used less commonly to assess clinical competence.

Where should the student be assessed?

Traditionally students have been assessed in an examination hall environment, using written papers or by formal clinical examinations in the hospital ward. With moves towards greater authenticity in assessment, and with assessment seen more as a continuous process, increased attention is being focused on assessment in the workplace and in the wide range of contexts where teaching takes place. This can be in the hospital or community environment.

Over to you

Reflect and React

1. Assessment is frequently one of the last things considered when a curriculum is planned. It is often the first thing the learner thinks about. Have you spent enough time considering the assessment of the learners in your programme?
2. From the list of purposes given above, what purposes are served by the examinations in your programme?
3. How would you rate your examination against the criteria given for a 'good assessment' and what learning outcomes are assessed?
4. Consider the use of a progress test.

Explore further

Journal articles

Fitzgerald, J.T., Burkhardt, J.C., Kasten, S.J., et al., 2015. Assessment challenges in competency-based education: a case study in health professions education. Med. Teach. [Epub ahead of print].
A description of competency-based assessment in the Master in Health Professions Education programme at the University of Michigan Medical School.
Harden, R., 2009. Five myths and the case against a European or national licensing examination. Med. Teach. 31, 217–220.
Hodges, B.D., Ginsburg, S., Cruess, R., et al., 2011. Assessment of professionalism: recommendations from the Ottawa 2010 conference. Med. Teach. 33, 354–363.

Holmboe, E.S., Batalden, P., 2015. Achieving the desired transformation: thoughts on next steps for outcome-based medical education. Acad. Med. 90, 1215–1223.
In outcome-based education, assessment is important.
Holmboe, E.S., Sherbino, J., Long, D.M., et al., 2010. The role of assessment in competency-based medical education. Med. Teach. 32, 676–682.
A competency-based approach to medical education relies on continuous, comprehensive, and elaborate assessment and feedback systems.
McGaghie, W.C., Barsuk, J.H., Wayne, D.B., 2015. Mastery learning with deliberate

practice in medical education. Acad. Med. 90 (11), 1575.

Norcini, J., Anderson, B., Bollela, V., 2011. Criteria for good assessment: consensus statement and recommendations from the Ottawa 2010 conference. Med. Teach. 33, 206–214.

Schuwirth, L.W.T., van der Vleuten, C.P.M., 2012. The use of progress testing. Perspect. Med. Educ. 1, 24–30.

Van der Vleuten, C.P., Schuwirth, L.W., 2005. Assessing professional competence: from methods to programmes. Med. Educ. 39, 309–317.
An introduction to programmatic assessment.

Van der Vleuten, C.P.M., Schuwirth, L.W.T., Driessen, E.W., et al., 2015. Twelve tips for programmatic assessment. Med. Teach. 37, 641–646.

Guides

Bandaranayake, R.C., 2010. Setting and Maintaining Standards in Multiple Choice Examinations. AMEE Guide No. 37. AMEE, Dundee.

McKinley, D.W., Norcini, J.J., 2014. How to set standards on performance-based examinations. AMEE Guide No. 85. Med. Teach. 36, 97–110.

Pangaro, L., ten Cate, O., 2013. Frameworks for learner assessment in medicine: AMEE Guide No. 78. Med. Teach. 35, e1197–e1210.

Schuwirth, L.W., van der Vleuten, C.P.M., 2011. General overview of the theories used in assessment: AMEE Guide No. 57. Med. Teach. 33, 783–797.

Shumway, J.M., Harden, R.M., 2003. The assessment of learning outcomes for the competent and reflective physicians. AMEE Medical Education Guide No. 25. Med. Teach. 25, 569–584.
A description of the assessment tools that can be used to assess the different outcomes of learning.

Wrigley, W., van der Vleuten, C.P.M., Freeman, A., et al., 2012. A systematic framework for the progress test: strengths, constraints and issues: AMEE Guide No. 71. Med. Teach. 34, 683–697.
This guide provides a framework for improving the quality and defensibility of progress test data.

Books

Downing, S.M., Yudkowsky, R. (Eds.), 2009. Assessment in Health Professions Education. Routledge, New York.

Harden, R.M., Lilley, P., Patricio, M., 2016. The Definitive Guide to the OSCE. Elsevier. Churchill, Livingstone.

Larsen, D.P., Butler, A.C., 2013. Test-enhanced learning. In: Walsh, K. (Ed.), Oxford Textbook of Medical Education. Oxford University Press, Oxford. (Chapter 38).

Written and computer-based assessment 31

Written questions have a role to play alongside other assessment methods.

Written assessment has a role to play

Written approaches to assessment are well established and are widely used to assess learners' competence in all spheres of education. In medical education written assessment is used to determine whether the learner has acquired the expected level of knowledge and can apply it to clinical problems. Despite the greater emphasis being placed on performance assessment, written approaches still have an important role to play as an instrument in the assessor's tool kit.

The use of written examinations has come under scrutiny with regard to their match with the expected learning outcomes and their impact on the learner's behaviour. What is assessed, however, is determined by the quality and construction of the question. There needs to be a balance between reliability and validity as described in Chapter 30 and different written assessment methods have been developed as a response to these challenges. Increasingly computers have replaced paper and pencil techniques for the delivery of the assessment.

The elements in a written assessment

It is helpful to think of written assessment in terms of the stimulus or task that necessitates a learner's response, the response itself and the assessment of it.

The stimulus

The stimulus for the learner's response may be:

- A question or short statement, e.g. 'In which of the following pathologies does a patient typically present with weight loss and an increased appetite?' or 'List the three options in the management of a patient with hyperthyroidism.'
- A statement or a question with accompanying diagrams or charts, e.g. 'In the diagram which structure is labelled "A"?'

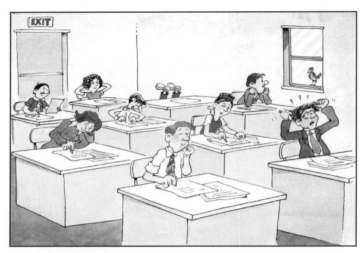

Figure 31.1 A written examination

- A short clinical scenario with a patient's presentation followed by a question, e.g. 'Mrs Wilkie, a 35-year-old waitress complaining of tiredness and nervousness … what is the most likely diagnosis?'
- A more extended patient management problem that develops over a period of time.

The student's response

The response expected of the learner can be categorised into:

- Constructed response or production questions, where the student has to write a long or short narrative in response to the stimulus. These include essays, short essay questions and short answer questions. They relate more closely to medical practice than multiple choice questions (MCQs). A patient does not present to the doctor with a list of five possible diagnoses. Short answer questions have been used successfully in progress tests and can better assess core knowledge without undue prompting, e.g. 'Which hormones are secreted by the thyroid gland?'
- Selected response or recognition questions, where the student has to make a selection from a range of options provided. These include MCQs, for example the one best answer or multiple true/false questions and extended matching questions (EMQs).

The assessment of a student's response

The student's response may be scored:

- Automatically by a computer as correct or incorrect, as in an MCQ where there is an agreed correct answer. This also applies to short answer questions where the expected answer is limited to a few words. In this case, agreement has to be reached with regard to alternative wording and spelling that is acceptable.

- By an examiner in a constructed response question, based on a holistic impression of the student's response, or with an agreed structured marking scheme.
- According to the answers to the questions provided by members of a panel of experts. This strategy is used in the script concordance test as described below.

Standard setting

A range of methods have been used in a written examination to determine the mark above which students will pass the examination and below which they will fail (Bandaranayake 2008).

It is not uncommon for a pass mark for an MCQ paper to be set at 60–70%. This implies, however, that students need to know only two-thirds of the area covered and that it does not matter which third they do not know. Although it is not usual practice, consideration needs to be given to an examination or part of an examination that assesses essential core knowledge, with a pass mark of more than 90% expected for that part of the examination. This is consistent with assessment for mastery learning as referred to in Chapter 30.

Types of written assessment

Essay questions

While the essay remains a common assessment tool in many fields, it is less commonly used in medicine. Provided the question or stimulus is appropriate, the essay can test:

- the learner's general understanding of the topic
- higher-level skills, including synthesis, organisation of information, analysis, problem solving and evaluation
- written communication skills, a competence often not tested by other written assessment methods although portfolio assessment may be used for this purpose
- aspects relating to attitudes and medical ethics.

However, essay questions have disadvantages as an assessment tool:

- the content area sampled is small compared to an MCQ paper
- the scoring of the questions is subjective and time consuming.

Short essay questions (SEQs)

Short essay questions are designed to sample a wider range of content than the essay question. A student may have to answer twelve 10-minute SEQs instead of four

30-minute or two 1-hour essay questions. The SEQ has many of the advantages and disadvantages of the essay question.

Short answer questions (SAQs)

In a short answer question, the student does not select from a list of choices as in a MCQ. Instead the student responds to the question in one, two or a limited number of words. The format has the advantages of an MCQ in that a wide range of content can be sampled and answers can be automatically marked using a computer program. Prior to this, agreement must be reached regarding 'acceptable' answers.

A significant advantage over MCQs is that the SAQ does not test simply recognition of the correct answer from a list of options. It is also easier to set questions that test core or basic knowledge without having to cue the learner with the responses on the list. SAQs merit wider consideration and adoption as an alternative to the MCQ.

Multiple choice questions (MCQs)

Multiple choice questions can sample objectively a wide range of a student's knowledge and understanding. The downside for the examiner is not the marking of the responses but the setting of the questions, which requires skill and effort. Several question banks have been developed in medicine and these allow schools to share questions.

Many MCQ examinations test mainly recall of knowledge rather than in-depth understanding or application. This has had a detrimental effect on how students study. To counteract this, there has been a move to introduce greater authenticity to the MCQ through the use of clinical scenarios in the stem or stimulus.

Many formats for MCQs have been described but two approaches have dominated:

- Single best option, where the learner is required to select the best response from four or five alternatives.
- Multiple true/false questions, where the student has to categorise as true or false each of five statements relating to the stem. Guessing is a more important consideration with this type of question and as a result the marking scheme may be more complicated. Partly because of this there has been a move away from using this type of question. Its use, however, should not be abandoned as it can be used to test a wider range of knowledge. Also the questions are easier to set without the need for distractors, as in the single best option type of question.

Extended matching questions (EMQs)

The EMQ is a type of written question in the selected response category that provides an alternative to the standard MCQ. The EMQ consists of a list of about twenty options relating to a theme or topic. This may be a list of drugs, diseases, laboratory investigations, symptoms, explanations or pathologies. Following the lead-in stem or stimulus, usually in the form of a patient scenario, the student has to select the most appropriate answer from the list of options. One, two or more questions can use the same list of options. The advantage here is that the effect of cuing is minimised. The questions are also less time consuming to produce as several scenarios can use the same list of options. As with MCQs, a computer can be used to score the answers.

The EMQ is a useful way of testing clinically relevant knowledge.

Modified essay questions (MEQs)

The MEQ is a sequence of questions based on a patient scenario that develops over a period of time. After the first question is answered, further information is provided about the patient and this is followed by another question. The typical MEQ may have six or more questions and both SAQs and MCQs may be used. Because of difficulties in the preparation of the questions and difficulties with scoring, this format is now used less frequently.

Script concordance test (SCT)

This is a relatively new form of written assessment. Students are given a brief evolving patient scenario and asked to make judgements regarding diagnostic possibilities or management options. To allow decisions to be made that reflect medical practice, the student is given sufficient clinical detail but a certain amount of uncertainty, imprecision or incompleteness is deliberately built into each case in order to simulate real-life clinical situations. The learner is assessed on the amount of agreement or concordance between his or her response and that of a panel of experts. The approach may be useful in assessing a student's clinical reasoning.

Situational judgement tests (SJTs)

SJTs are a relatively new form of assessment question in medical education. They have been used for assessing students for admission to medicine, and assessing a doctor's entry to postgraduate training. The questions test whether the examinee responds to a real-life situation in an appropriate way, e.g. what should the junior doctor do if the consultant prescribes an incorrect dose of a drug, or how to respond to a patient with cancer who does not ask about the diagnosis. As the answers are usually in a MCQ format they can be easily marked. The preparation of the questions is not easy and experts may disagree about the answers.

The technology

Questions can be posed, responses recorded and examinations scored either on paper or on a computer. Computers are now widely used for MCQs: the students answer using a computer and their responses are automatically scored. There is also some interest in adaptive testing. This is when the questions posed on the computer are determined by the students' responses to earlier questions. A wrong answer to a question may generate additional related questions that allow the student's understanding or lack of understanding of the area to be explored further. This may increase the reliability of the examination by increasing the number of questions used in the areas where the student's understanding is in doubt. To date this approach is not routinely used.

Over to you

Reflect and react

1. Given the learning outcomes to be tested and the resources available, which format of written test is appropriate in your setting?
2. To what extent does a written examination in your course test more than factual recall?
3. Consider how you can best provide feedback to students about their performance in a written examination. Simply providing a mark, for example 62%, is not sufficient.

Exploring further

Journal articles

Amin, Z., Boulet, J.R., Cook, D.A., et al., 2011. Technology-enabled assessment of health professions education: consensus statement and recommendations from the Ottawa 2010 Conference. Med. Teach. 33, 364–369.

Kelly, W., Durning, W., Denton, G., 2012. Comparing a script concordance examination to a multiple-choice examination on a core internal medical clerkship. Teach. Learn. Med. J. 24, 187–193.

The script concordance examination was a more valid assessment in practice than the MCQ.

Rademakers, J., ten Cate, T.H.J., Bar, P.R., 2005. Progress testing with short answer questions. Med. Teach. 27, 578–582.

Schuwirth, L.W., van der Vleuten, C.P., 2004. Different written assessment methods: what can be said about their strengths and weaknesses? Med. Educ. 38, 974–979.

Guides

Bandaranayake, R.C., 2008. Setting and maintaining standards in multiple choice examinations. AMEE Guide No. 37. Med. Teach. 30, 836–845.

Lubarsky, S., Dory, V., Duggan, P., et al., 2013. Script concordance testing: from theory to practice. AMEE Guide No. 75. Med. Teach. 35, 184–193.

Books

Case, S.M., Swanson, D.B., 2002. Constructing Written Test Questions for the Basic and Clinical Sciences, third ed. (revised). National Board of Medical Examiners, Philadelphia.

A classic description of how to prepare MCQs.

Hayes, K., 2013. Written assessment. In: Walsh, K. (Ed.), Oxford Textbook of Medical Education. Oxford University Press, Oxford. (Chapter 47)

A description of the uses of the different types of written questions with examples of each type.

32

An assessment of a student's clinical competence is key to an assessment of their ability to practise medicine.

The importance of clinical assessment

Clinical and work-based assessment instruments assess the clinical and practical skills of examinees and how their knowledge is applied in the clinical context. The clinical examination is of key importance in the assessment of the learner's competence to practise medicine, and in many schools is the cornerstone in qualifying examinations. No one would want to fly in an aircraft where the pilot had been certified to fly based on his performance in a written examination with no practical assessment of his competence. It is the same for doctors. We expect them to have been assessed with regard to their practical skills before leaving medical school and certified that they have the necessary competencies to meet the needs of the patients for whom they will be responsible.

The assessment of competence can be distinguished from performance assessment. Tests of competence, such as the objective structured clinical examination (OSCE), demonstrate in a controlled situation what an examinee is capable of doing. Performance assessment tools, such as analysis of patient records or multi-source feedback, assess what the individual does in practice. Miller's pyramid provides a framework for assessment (Miller 1990), with the bottom of the pyramid being the assessment of knowledge and the higher levels of the pyramid being the assessment of performance (Figure 32.1).

The patient

Central to the clinical examination is the interaction between the examinee and a patient. For the purpose of the examination, the patient may be a 'real' patient, a simulated patient or a manikin or a computer representation used as a patient substitute. In the clinical examination there are benefits in using a range of patient representations. The choice will be influenced by what is being assessed, the required level of standardisation, the desired realism or fidelity and the local logistics. These include the availability and relative costs associated with the use of real patients and trained simulated patients (Collins and Harden 1998).

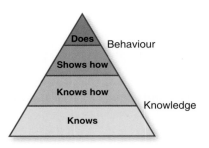

Figure 32.1 Miller's pyramid of clinical competence (Miller 1990)

'Real' patients

The traditional clinical examination was based on 'real' patients. 'Real' patients are widely used in OSCE situations although this is less common in North America. The organisers of the examination may have access to a bank of patients with a range of pathologies such as a patient with goitre, rheumatoid arthritis or hemiplegia. 'Real' patients are the basis for the patient encounter in work-based assessment.

Simulated patients

Difficulties in standardising real patients and a lack of availability in some situations led to the development of simulated or standardised patients. These have been used for assessment as well as teaching. The simulated patient, as described in Chapter 27, is usually a lay person who has undergone various levels of training in order to provide a consistent clinical scenario. The examinee interacts with the simulated patient in the same way as if they were taking a history, examining or counselling a real patient. Simulated patients are used most commonly to assess history taking and communication skills or physical examination where no abnormality is found. Simulated patients have also been used to simulate a range of physical findings, for example, different neurological presentations. The term 'standardised patient' has been used to indicate that the person has been trained to play the role of the patient consistently and according to specific criteria.

Simulators and models

Simulators, from the very basic models used to assess skills such as skin suturing to the more complex interactive whole-body manikins such as SimMan, have been used increasingly in medical training as outlined in Chapter 27. They have an important role to play in assessment. The Harvey cardiac manikin has been used at an OSCE station to assess skills in cardiac auscultation. Simulators can also be used to assess procedural and practical skills, including the insertion of intravenous lines, catheterisation and endoscopy technique. While simulators have played a key role in competence assessment in other fields, notably with airline pilots, they were slow to have an impact in the area of assessment in medicine. The situation has changed rapidly and such devices now play a prominent role in clinical assessment. Indeed, in some instances surgeons are allowed to perform a procedure in clinical practice only after they have demonstrated competence on a simulator.

Computer-based simulations

The development of virtual patients is another area where rapid progress is being made. While early computer-based simulations were little more than patient management problems delivered through a computer, computer simulations now include high-fidelity models of the patient care environment and the 'patient' responds to the management and therapeutic efforts of the examinee.

Approaches to clinical and performance assessment

A range of methods have been used to assess the student's or trainee's competence in a controlled clinical environment and to assess how they perform in the workplace or real clinical situation.

The objective structured long examination record (OSLER)

In the traditional long case, the examinee takes a history and examines the patient over a period of up to an hour unobserved by the examiner. The examiner then meets with the student and over a 20–30 minute period discusses the patient and the examinee's findings and conclusions. The OSLER was proposed to replace the 'long case' component of a clinical examination, as being a more objective and valid assessment of the student's clinical competence (Gleeson 1997).

Over a 30-minute period the examiner uses a structured score sheet to assess the examinee's performance with a patient in the following areas:

- history taking scored in relation to pace and clarity of presentation, communication skills, systematic approach and the establishment of the case facts
- physical examination rated in relation to a systematic approach, examination technique and the establishment of the correct physical findings
- the ability to determine appropriate investigations for the patient
- the examinee's views on the management of the patient
- the clinical acumen and overall ability to identify and present a satisfactory approach to tackling the patient's problems.

The examiner grades the examinee's performance for each of the areas assessed, taking into account the difficulty of the case, with a rating of 'excellent', 'very good', 'pass', 'bare pass', 'below pass' or 'seriously below pass'. The examiner also records an overall grade for the complete performance.

The objective structured clinical examination (OSCE)

The OSCE was introduced in 1975 in response to criticisms about the reliability and validity of the traditional clinical examination. It has been adopted worldwide and is now recognised as the gold standard for the assessment of clinical competence (Harden et al. 2015). Students rotate around a series of stations at a predetermined time interval. Each station focuses on one or more aspects of competence, such as history taking, physical examination or carrying out a procedure. An OSCE can include 'real', simulated or standardised patients, manikins and simulators. Each has advantages in what they can offer for the purpose of the assessment. Such a mixture is not always possible and 'real' patients or simulated patients may dominate the OSCE.

While the details vary, a typical OSCE lasts two hours and has 24 stations with 5 minutes allocated for each station. This allows a wide sample of competencies to be assessed. Some OSCEs have fewer stations with a longer time allotted for each station. In general, however, it is preferable to use more, shorter stations rather than longer ones as this increases the reliability and validity of the examination. An OSCE with twenty-four 5-minute stations is preferable to an examination with twelve 10-minute stations.

If a task cannot be completed in the 5-minute period there are three options:

• The task can be revised so that it can be completed in 5 minutes.
• The task can be spread across two linked stations. The first part of the task, for example assessing a patient's record, can be undertaken at the first station, and the subsequent task of counselling the patient assessed at the following station.
• A station may be duplicated in the circuit to allow students to spend double the set time at the station. This may be useful for a history taking station.

In the OSCE, any subjective bias attributed to an examiner is reduced as the student will encounter a number of examiners during the course of the examination. What is assessed at each station is agreed in advance and a marking schedule is produced which is completed by the examiner. It is important that examiners are fully briefed and trained in advance. Examples of the types of stations that can be included in an OSCE are given in Appendix 9.

The OSCE offers major attractions as a reliable and valid test of clinical competence. In addition, because of its adaptability, it can be modified to meet local needs, including what is assessed, the role of examiners, the duration and number of stations (Harden et al. 2015).

Mini clinical evaluation exercise (Mini-CEX)

In a Mini-CEX the examinee is engaged in an authentic workplace-based patient encounter. This may be in the outpatient department, the inpatient setting or emergency room. The examiner watches the examinee take a focused history, perform relevant parts of the physical examination, provide a diagnosis and present a management plan. The encounter usually lasts about 15–20 minutes and the examiner spends 5 minutes giving the examinee feedback. The performance is scored on a 6- or 9-point scale ranging from below expectations through borderline and meeting expectations to above expectations. The examinee is responsible for the timing of the encounter and for the selection of the patient. The Mini-CEX is repeated on a number of occasions during a clinical attachment with different examiners and different patients.

The Mini-CEX was developed for use in a postgraduate setting but it has been used also in undergraduate education. In this situation the duration of the encounter is often increased from 20 to 40 minutes.

The Mini-CEX has the advantage that it ensures that the clinical skills of the student or trainee are observed by the clinician or trainer in the workplace setting and that feedback is given to the learner. The briefing of the examiner and examinee are important.

Direct observation of procedural skills (DOPS)

This is a variation of the Mini-CEX designed to assess and give feedback on a student's or trainee's procedural skills. As in the Mini-CEX the student or trainee is observed in the workplace carrying out the procedure on 'real' patients. The trainee selects the timing and the procedure to be assessed from a prescribed list, including, for example, central venous line insertion, arterial blood sampling, electrocardiography and intubation. The examiner may be a clinician or another member of the healthcare team. As with the Mini-CEX, DOPS was designed for use in postgraduate education but has also been applied in undergraduate education.

Case-based discussion (CbD)

The CbD is used principally in postgraduate training. The trainee selects several case records in which they have made entries regarding patients they have seen recently. The examiner selects one patient record and explores aspects of it with the trainee. The assessment is designed to assess application of knowledge, decision making and ethical issues as well as medical record keeping. Dimensions assessed include the trainee's clinical assessment of the patient, investigations and referrals, treatment, follow-up and future planning, professionalism and overall clinical judgement. Each dimension is scored on a 6-point scale. Fifteen minutes is allowed for the examination followed by 5 minutes' feedback.

Multi-source feedback (MSF) or 360 degrees evaluation

MSF has been used for many years in industry and has been adopted for use in medicine. It is used mainly in postgraduate and continuing education to assess the practising doctor but can also be used in undergraduate education. Evidence is collected systematically from a number of individuals who are in a legitimate position to make a judgement about the doctor's or student's performance. The individuals may be senior or junior colleagues, other members of the healthcare team, administrators, patients or students. In this way, different perspectives are brought to bear on the evaluation of the doctor. Each individual is asked to complete a structured questionnaire relating to the doctor's performance. A rating scale of '1 to 5' or '1 to 7' can be used and comments may also be recorded. The questions asked may be the same or vary for different groups of respondents. Information is collated so that the ratings remain anonymous and the results are fed back to the doctor. The aim is to provide a fair and balanced view of the doctor's behaviour and abilities, particularly in areas such as communication skills, leadership, team working, punctuality and reliability. MSF is less frequently used in undergraduate education but is sometimes included for assessment purposes in a student's portfolio. This may include peer assessment of professionalism.

MSF offers many advantages, in particular the assessment of the doctor in the real-life practice context. It also has potential disadvantages, in particular the risk of providing damaging and over-harsh feedback.

A portfolio

A portfolio can be used in the assessment of a student's or trainee's competence, as described in Chapter 33.

Implementing a clinical assessment

The assessment of a student's clinical competence is a major responsibility for a teacher. It requires careful planning and execution.

A blueprint

A blueprint or grid should be prepared that includes the competencies or learning outcomes to be assessed. For each outcome, note the assessment method to be adopted.

Selection of methods

A range of methods should be used. Some will be snapshots at a particular point in time, such as an OSCE or a Mini-CEX; others will be based on evidence collected over a period of time, e.g. a portfolio.

A programmatic approach, as described in Chapter 30, is valuable, with decisions about a student's competence in a domain based on the triangulation of evidence from a number of sources. This is of particular importance in a domain such as attitudes, professionalism or empathy.

The examiner

The examiner has an important role to play. This includes the collection of evidence about the examinee's behaviour in the context of the assessment and based on this, passing judgement on the examinee's competence or performance. The examiner may be a clinician or another healthcare professional. Simulated patients, after appropriate training, are used in some situations, particularly in North America, to assess the student's performance in an OSCE. Patients and other members of the healthcare team frequently contribute to multi-source feedback assessment. Whatever the assessment method used, it is important to include a number of examiners.

A problem with the long case in the traditional clinical examination was overreliance on the ratings of one or two examiners. In contrast, the OSCE has input from a number of examiners, which is a major advantage and contributes to its reliability.

A student's profile

A wide range of different learning outcomes or competencies are assessed in a clinical examination. These include clinical skills, practical procedures, clinical reasoning, decision making, problem solving, collaboration, team working, professionalism and attitudes. It makes little sense simply to allocate a percentage score for each component and then to sum these to produce a total mark for the examination, for example, 62%. Excellence in carrying out a physical examination of a patient or practical procedure should not compensate for unprofessional behaviour or an inappropriate attitude. Do not agonise over the relative importance of each element of competence and the allocation of a percentage for that element. It is best to produce a competence profile for the examinee. This indicates for each candidate, as shown in Figure 32.2, the domains where their performance is satisfactory and meets the standard expected or is perhaps excellent, and also those domains or competencies where the candidate's performance falls short of what is expected.

Feedback

Providing feedback to the examinee is an important part of a clinical assessment. As discussed in Chapter 3, this should be specific and timely. Feedback is an essential element and plays an important part when assessment is being used as a tool for learning ('assessment for learning'), and guiding learners in their further studies. When the assessment process is planned, it is important that time is allowed for the provision of feedback. The OSCE can be considered as an example of the different feedback approaches that can be adopted (Harden et al. 2015):

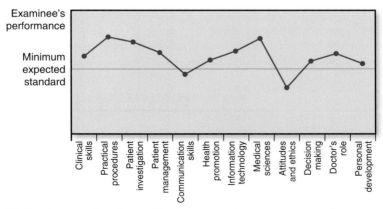

Figure 32.2 An examinee's profile demonstrating competence in some areas but not others

1. During an OSCE, time is allocated at the end of each station to allow the examiner to give feedback to the examinee.
2. Immediately after completion of an OSCE station, the examinees review their performance at the next station using the examiner's checklist and a video recording of a model performance.
3. Following an OSCE, the checklists and ratings sheets for each station with the examiner's comments can be returned to the examinee.
4. Following an OSCE, teachers meet with individuals or with the whole class to discuss the examination.
5. The candidate is given the opportunity to watch a video recording of his or her performance, and compare it to an example of what was expected.

Over to you

Reflect and react

1. The assessment of a student's clinical competence is of the greatest importance. Whatever your role as a teacher, you should be aware of the different approaches and tools available.
2. Prepare a blueprint or grid relating the learning outcomes in your programme to the different assessment methods.
3. You may have to serve as an examiner in an OSCE or be the person responsible for providing students with feedback on their performance. Your role may be to advise students or trainees how to prepare for the examination. Ensure that you are familiar with the examination details.
4. Assessment of the doctor's performance in the workplace is particularly challenging. The examiner and examinee both need to be committed to its success. Think about how you might distinguish between your trainees' competence and performance.

Explore further

Journal articles

Boursicot, K., Etheridge, L., Setna, Z., et al., 2011. Performance in assessment: consensus statement and recommendations from the Ottawa Conference. Med. Teach. 33, 370–383.

Harden, R.M., 2015. Misconceptions and the OSCE. Med. Teach. [in press].

Hill, F., Kendall, K., 2007. Adopting and adapting the mini-CEX as an undergraduate assessment and learning tool. Clin. Teach. 4, 244–248.
How the Mini-CEX can be used in undergraduate education.

Miller, G.E., 1990. The assessment of clinical skills/competence/performance. Acad. Med. 65, S63–S67.

Guides

Collins, J.P., Harden, R.M., 1998. The use of real patients, simulated patients and simulators in clinical examinations. AMEE Medical Education Guide No. 13. Med. Teach. 20, 508–521.

Gleeson, F., 1997. Assessment of clinical competence using the Objective Structured Long Examination Record (OSLER). AMEE Medical Education Guide No. 9. Med. Teach. 19, 7–14.

Harden, R.M., 2015. Revisiting 'Assessment of clinical competence using an objective structured clinical examination (OSCE)'. Med. Educ. [in press].
A historical perspective on the OSCE.

Harden, R.M., Gleeson, F.A., 1979. Assessment of medical competence using an objective structured clinical examination (OSCE). Med. Educ. 13, 41–54.

An early description of the OSCE but still with much relevance today.

Norcini, J., Burch, V., 2007. Work-place Based Assessment as an Educational Tool. AMEE Medical Education Guide No. 31. AMEE, Dundee.

Books

Harden, R.M., Lilley, P., Patricio, M., 2015. The Definitive Guide to the OSCE. Elsevier, London.

Holmboe, E.S., Hawkins, R.E., 2008. Practical Guide to the Evaluation of Clinical Competence. Mosby, St Louis.

Norcini, J., Holmboe, E., 2010. Work-based assessment. In: Cantillon, P., Wood, D. (Eds.), ABC of Learning and Teaching in Medicine, second ed. Wiley–Blackwell, Chichester. (Chapter 11).

Tekian, A., McGuire, C.H., McGaghie, W.C., 1999. Innovative Simulations for Assessing Professional Competence: From Paper-and-Pencil to Virtual Reality. University of Illinois at Chicago Department of Medical Education.

CLINICAL AND PERFORMANCE-BASED ASSESSMENT

The use of a portfolio for assessment purposes is a response to changes in medical education, including the emphasis on professionalism and the need to give students more responsibility for their own learning.

What is a portfolio?

A portfolio is a collection of evidence demonstrating that learning has taken place. It is cumulative in the sense that it contains work collected over a period of time rather than the snapshot view obtained with the traditional examination. Portfolios have been used in the arts for many years, and now have a major impact as an assessment tool in medicine and other healthcare professions. Portfolios are an authentic learning and assessment tool that relates to the work of a doctor and reflects a holistic and integrated approach to medical practice. It is important to appreciate that a portfolio is different from a logbook. In a portfolio the learner's experiences and reflections are recorded together with a description of the further learning that has resulted.

The portfolio is likely to contain both quantitative graded evidence as well as qualitative descriptions. Students actively collect and select material for their portfolio which will provide the examiner with evidence of their learning. Portfolios may include evidence of the practical procedures carried out by the student, video records of their clinical experiences, evaluations of their performance in written assessments and reports by clinicians on the student's clinical attachments. Multi-source feedback from nurses, other members of the healthcare team and patients may be included. The students individualise their portfolio by selecting the evidence relating to their own personal experience. The nature of the evidence is limited only by the degree of the student's creativity.

Why portfolios?

In the 1970s, as described in Chapter 32, there was a switch of emphasis from an assessment of students' knowledge to an assessment of their clinical skills, including history taking, physical examination and practical procedures. Tools such as the objective structured clinical examination (OSCE) were developed for this purpose. The more recent move to outcome-based education with an emphasis on learning outcomes such as attitudes, professionalism, reflection and self-assessment created the need for a tool that provided a valid assessment in these areas. There was a need too for an assessment tool that counteracted a reductionist approach to assessment and which provided a more holistic and overall assessment of a student's competence.

My (RMH) daughter completed two honours degree courses. One was in mathematics and computing and the other in fashion design. She was in no doubt that the assessment method used in her fashion course – a portfolio assessment – was a much more searching, reliable, valid and fairer assessment of her competence in a professional area than the more traditional examinations used in the mathematics and computing course. Her fashion portfolio provided evidence of work completed during her studies and her reflections on this. It included evidence of the technical and interpersonal skills she had acquired during her training and demonstrated her understanding of the theory that underpinned the work. Her experience illustrated the potential value of a portfolio as an assessment tool and its relevance to medicine was apparent.

Advantages

Portfolios offer a number of advantages as an assessment tool:

- Portfolios can be used to assess outcomes and competencies where other tools have been less successful. These may be skills necessary for lifelong learning such as self-assessment, reflection and the adoption of appropriate learning strategies. The portfolio is a tool that contributes to the assessment of a student's attitudes and professionalism.
- Portfolios include evidence collected over a period of time and provide an overall and holistic view of a student's competence.
- Portfolios can include a range of quantitative and qualitative evidence. With triangulation of the different sources of evidence, portfolios support the examiner in making a comprehensive and reliable interpretation of a student's achievement.
- Portfolios represent a personalised approach to assessment that focuses more on what individual students achieve rather than the more standardised approach with instruments such as the OSCE.
- The portfolio is a powerful tool for both learning and assessment. As the students go through their course of studies the portfolio focuses the student's attention on the learning outcomes expected and integrates learning and assessment. In the later years the student's reflection on the basic sciences relevant to documented patient encounters reinforces the application of basic sciences to clinical practice.
- The portfolio reinforces a student-centred approach to the curriculum, with students being given greater responsibility for their own learning.

Implementing portfolio assessment in practice

The late Miriam Friedman Ben-David described the following steps in the portfolio assessment process to aid those wishing to design and implement portfolio assessment in their own institution (Friedman Ben-David et al. 2001):

1. **Define the purpose.** It should be made clear whether the portfolio is to be used for summative or formative decisions and how it relates to other elements in the assessment process.
2. **Determine the competencies to be assessed.** Identifying the competencies to be assessed by the portfolio is part of a systematic approach to assessment that ensures that all of the expected learning outcomes are assessed. In particular, the portfolio is valuable in assessing learning outcomes such as attitudes and professionalism, and the higher levels of Miller's pyramid (see Chapter 32).
3. **Define the portfolio content.** Evidence should be included in the portfolio that demonstrates a student's achievement of the learning outcomes to be assessed. Students should be given guidelines about the type of evidence that is acceptable, but there should be a certain amount of freedom of choice. The type of evidence that is included, the student's comments on it and the student's ability to assess their own competence is a measure of their understanding of the learning outcomes and their self-assessment skills. Examples of the type of evidence that might be included are:
   - records of procedures carried out by the student
   - annotated details of patient encounters with details of how they contributed to the student's achievement of the learning outcomes
   - video recordings of the student's interaction with patients
   - evaluation of the student during clinical clerkships by members of the healthcare team, including nurses and patients
   - results of the student's performance in formal assessments, including OSCEs and written assessments
   - in the case of a practising doctor, a dossier of evidence demonstrating the doctor's continuing education and practice achievements. The evidence included in a portfolio should indicate the student's or practising doctor's progress over time.
4. **Develop a marking system.** For each of the learning outcomes to be assessed with the portfolio, specific criteria should be set out and a global rating used for the achievement of each outcome:
   4 – excellent, distinguished or superior
   3 – satisfactory, adequate or competent
   2 – minimal, borderline or marginal
   1 – unsatisfactory or inadequate
5. **Select and train the examiners.** Several assessors should review each portfolio with an assessment committee taking a final decision. The choice of examiners will depend on the purpose of the assessment and the learning outcomes to be assessed. The examiners should include a range of staff from the basic sciences and clinical medicine. Examiners with less experience can

be paired with more senior examiners. The training of the examiners is essential for the success of the programme. Faculty members often welcome their participation in portfolio examinations as it allows them to get to know more about the individual student and their capabilities.

6. **Plan the examination process and timetable**. A deadline should be set for portfolio submissions. Students' failure to meet the deadline is itself evidence of a lack of professionalism. Time should be scheduled for examiners to read each portfolio and meet to discuss them with co-examiners. An examiner should then meet, possibly in pairs, with each student to allow the student to defend the portfolio. Finally time needs to be set aside for the examiners to discuss each student's performance in order to reach a final decision on the student's achievement of the learning outcomes assessed.

7. **Student orientation**. Students should be informed in writing about the portfolio assessment process and what is expected of them. In general, the more information given to students the more positive they are about the portfolio.

8. **Develop guidelines for decisions**. If portfolios are used for summative pass/ fail decisions, standards need to be specified so that there is no doubt about what constitutes a pass or a fail. A decision needs to be made whether poor performance in relation to one outcome can be compensated by good or excellent performance in another area, or whether areas are not compensatory. The medical school in Dundee adopted the approach that a student cannot compensate for deficits in a key domain, such as attitudes or professionalism, by a good performance in another domain. Students must achieve the minimum expected standard in every domain.

Over to you

Reflect and react

1. Review the value of portfolios as a tool for student assessment. Which of the advantages listed are applicable to the programme for which you have a responsibility?
2. What learning outcomes can best be assessed by a portfolio?
3. What could be included in your student's or trainee's portfolio that would provide evidence of their achievement of the expected learning outcomes?
4. If you are an examiner for a portfolio assessment it is important that you fully understand the assessment process and the marking scheme used.

Explore further

Journal articles

Davis, M.H., Friedman Ben-David, M., Harden, R.M., et al., 2001. Portfolio assessment in medical students' final examinations. Med. Teach. 23, 357–366.

Driessen, E., van Tartwijk, J., van der Vleuten, C., et al., 2007. Portfolios in medical education: why do they meet with mixed success? A systematic review. Med. Educ. 41, 1224–1233.

Guides

Buckley, S., Coleman, J., Davidson, I., et al., 2009. The educational effects of portfolios on undergraduate student learning: BEME Guide No. 11. Med. Teach. 31, 282–298.

Friedman Ben-David, M., Davis, M.H., Harden, R.M., et al., 2001. Portfolios as a Method of Student Assessment. AMEE Medical Education Guide No. 24. AMEE, Dundee.

Tochel, C., Haig, A., Hesketh, A., et al., 2009. The effectiveness of portfolios for postgraduate assessment and education. BEME Guide No. 12. Med. Teach. 31, 299–318.

van Tartwijk, J., Driessen, E.W., 2010. Portfolios for Assessment and Learning. AMEE Guide No. 45. AMEE, Dundee.

Assessment for admission to medicine and postgraduate training 34

A range of assessment tools and approaches are available to assist with key selection decisions.

The importance of selection

Students can be selected and admitted to medical studies directly on leaving school or following another university course. The selection is important and for a number of reasons noted below is the focus of attention of the stakeholders, who include the potential students, their parents, the public, the government and the medical profession.

- With low attrition rates, the admission of a student to medical school is almost equivalent to graduating a student. Once students are selected for admission they will almost certainly complete their medical studies and graduate as a doctor.
- The criteria used for selection were based traditionally on academic qualifications. It was assumed that if a student achieved top grades at school they would automatically develop the competencies expected of a good doctor at medical school. This is not necessarily true. The personal qualities of the potential doctor are recognised to be important as well as their academic qualifications. How we train our doctors is of great importance, but what sort of doctor we produce will be determined to a large extent by the students we select for admission.
- Errors and inappropriate behaviour by doctors in clinical practice have attracted adverse problems and concern has been expressed that students are admitted to study medicine who may be unsuitable to practise as a doctor.
- The geographical origin of the student selected matters, as once students graduate they are more likely to practise in the geographical area or type of community where they originally lived.
- There is a need to increase the diversity of doctors trained so that they more closely match the needs of the community they will serve. Some ethnic and social classes may have been disadvantaged by the selection process and this needs to be taken into consideration.

Graduate or direct from school entry

In North America, following the Flexner 1910 Report, students were admitted to medical school as graduates following completion of a college course in another subject. In other parts of the world students can enter medical studies direct from school. There has been a move in some medical schools in the UK, Australia and other countries to graduate-only entry. At the same time there has also been a move in some schools in the United States to successfully shorten the time required in medical training by truncating the premedical course.

Some schools have maintained a mixed approach, accepting both graduates and school leavers. The issue is a controversial one and the arguments for the different approaches are complex. There is no good evidence to indicate that one approach is preferable to the other, but opting to admit students straight from school does have significant financial advantages and there is no evidence that the quality of the product (the doctors produced) is less satisfactory.

Aims of selection

The aims of selection are:

- To admit students or trainees who will complete their studies or training programme. Many studies of selection methods have used this as a measure of the success and predictive validity of the education approach adopted.
- To graduate doctors or specialists who are best equipped to meet the needs of the community they will serve.

Criteria for selection methods

There are a wide variety of approaches to selecting students for admission to medical studies or a trainee for specialist training. The criteria for choosing a selection method are similar to those for any assessment.

- **Is the method valid?** Does it measure what it should measure? In the past, and still in many schools today, selection is based on academic excellence as judged by past academic performance at school or university. Individuals are selected who will do well in the medical school examinations rather than individuals who have the personal qualities to become a competent and good doctor. The ability to perform well in tests may simply predict later test scores and not performance as a doctor. The ability to answer MCQs correctly does not necessarily indicate that a student will be a good doctor. This does not mean that a choice has to be made between someone who has a good academic record and someone who has the personal qualities to become a good doctor. They are not mutually exclusive. When examining the validity of the selection method the question should also be asked whether the method contributes to the aim of broadening access to medical studies.

- **Is the method reliable?** During the selection process evidence should be collected from a range of sources.
- **Is it feasible or practical?** This is an important consideration given the number of applicants and the expense of implementing some of the selection approaches. A two-stage process may be adopted whereby applicants are initially screened on the basis of their academic achievement and a smaller cohort selected where the final decision is made on an assessment of personal qualities.
- **Is it acceptable?** It is important that the selection process is transparent and that the approach adopted is acceptable to students, their parents, the medical school and the public at large.
- **What is the impact?** The choice of selection method may determine, for example, which students apply to study medicine and may encourage a wider diversity among applicants.

Selection for admission differs from other assessments of students previously discussed. The aim is to identify a set number of students who will be admitted (and who meet the criteria) in line with the number of places available rather than to identify all who meet the set criteria. Some students who could potentially become good doctors will not be accepted.

Choice of method

Methods should be adopted that assess the applicants' academic, cognitive abilities and their personal qualities. The qualities looked for in the candidate for admission should take into account the specified learning outcomes of the school and the expected starting point or minimum requirement for each of the domains described in Chapter 10. This may include, for example, communication skills, attitudes, team skills, problem solving and creativity. To achieve this, a range of methods will be required.

Academic record and performance at school

Academic achievement and performance at school, as evidenced, for example, by A-level achievements in the UK or grade point averages (GPAs) in the United States, have played a major role in decisions about selection. Correlations have been shown between such indicators and students' performance in medical school, particularly in examinations in the early years.

Autobiographical narrative

A personal statement by the student may contain information about the applicant that will inform the admission decision. The student may be required to provide a narrative to justify their motivation to study medicine. Such descriptions, however, are at risk of plagiarism or fraud and may be written by a third party.

References

References may be sought from the student's school, previous employers or individuals with whom the student has been associated. Such letters of recommendation seek to identify personal qualities such as honesty and application. These references, however, have low validity, are open to bias and tend to be unreliable and ineffective. Laws in relation to disclosure and the removal of confidentiality cast additional doubt on their value. They may be of more value in identifying weak applicants who should not be admitted.

Interviews

Interviews have been widely used to complement the assessment of the student's achievement and aptitude and tend to be widely accepted by the public. While questions have been raised about their reliability, they are used to provide evidence that the student has some of the attitudes and attributes, such as communication skills, expected of a future doctor. Structured or semi-structured interviews, where the questions asked are standardised for the candidates and a rating scale is used, have been shown to be more reliable. Interviews, however, are labour-intensive and also subject to bias as the following example shows. In one school, when the measurements were taken for refurbishment of the bars in the student union it was found that the students previously admitted to the medical school were taller than average. A possible explanation was that the individual in charge of the interview admission process at that time was 6 feet 6 inches tall. When interviews are used, training of the interviewer is important.

The multiple mini-interview (MMI)

In recent years there has been increasing emphasis on more objective assessment of students for the purposes of selection with the use of an OSCE. The multiple mini-interview (MMI) consists of a series of 5- to 8-minute testing stations and has much to commend it as a selection tool. A rater at each station assesses the student's performance in areas such as ethical decision making, effective communication, empathy, manual dexterity, knowledge of the healthcare system and critical thinking. The MMI requires fewer examiner hours than the traditional type of interviews that involved a panel of examiners. The evidence to date is that the MMI has predictive validity. It provides also a stimulus to prompt admission committees to be more explicit about the qualities they are looking for in applicants.

General mental ability and aptitude tests

Various aptitude tests have been designed to measure a student's ability to develop skills or acquire knowledge. Most have a knowledge component. They measure overall performance against a range of mental abilities. Examples are the Medical College Admission Test (MCAT) in North America, the Graduate Australian Medical Admission Test (GAMAT), the United Kingdom Clinical Aptitude Test (UKCAT) and the BioMedical Admissions Test (BMAT).

Situational judgement tests (SJTs)

SJTs are used particularly in postgraduate trainee selection to assess the trainee's judgement regarding situations encountered in the workplace and what is effective behaviour in a given situation. The approach is discussed in Chapter 31.

Personality inventories

The use of personality tests as a selection tool in medicine has been controversial. The Personal Qualities Assessment tool has been developed in Australia as a battery of tests to assess moral orientation, resilience, self-control and involvement. Its use has been suggested as a method of excluding from medicine the small number of applicants who have undesirable non-academic personal qualities (Powis 2015).

Selection for admission to specialty training

Many of the issues concerning the selection of students to medical studies also apply to the selection of doctors for postgraduate training. Undergraduate performance and interviews play a significant part in the process. Dean's letters and other references are often used, but again their reliability is suspect.

Not much attention has been paid to matching doctors on graduation with the career for which they are best suited. The skills expected of a surgeon will differ in some respects from the abilities and characteristics expected of a doctor working in public health.

Over to you

Reflect and react

1. Familiarise yourself with the selection procedure in your institution. To what extent does it reflect the attributes expected of a future doctor?
2. To what extent do the principles of good assessment described above apply to the selection process in your institution?
3. If you are involved in a selection committee, an interview panel or as an assessor in an MMI you should ensure that you are familiar with the rules and complete the necessary training.
4. Consider how the social accountability of universities should be reflected in the student selection process and in widening access to medical training.

Explore further

Journal articles

Eva, K.W., Rosenfield, J., Reiter, H.I., et al., 2004. An admissions OSCE: the multiple mini-interview. Med. Educ. 38, 314–326.

Green, M.M., Welty, L., Thomas, J.X., et al., 2015. Academic performance of students in an accelerated baccalaureate/MD program: implications for alternative physician education pathways. Acad. Med. [In press].
A need to redefine medical student selection criteria.

Harris, S., Owen, C., 2007. Discerning quality: using the multiple mini-interview in student selection for the Australian National University Medical School. Med. Educ. 41, 234–241.

Powis, D., 2015. Selecting medical students: an unresolved challenge. Med. Teach. 37, 252–260.
Greater attention should be paid in selection to identifying unsuitable candidates using, for example, the Personal Qualities Assessment Tool.

Prideaux, D., Roberts, C., Eva, K., et al., 2011. Assessment for selection for the health care professions and specialty training: consensus statement and recommendations from the Ottawa 2010 conference. Med. Teach. 33, 215–223.

Books

Harden, R.M., Lilley, P., Patricio, M., 2015. A Definitive Guide to the OSCE. Elsevier, London.
A description of the OSCE and an example of a MMI.

McManus, C., 2013. Student selection. In: Dent, J., Harden, R.M. (Eds.), A Practical Guide for Medical Teachers. Elsevier, London (Chapter 43).

Patterson, F., 2013. Selection into medical education, training and practice. In: Walsh, K. (Ed.), Oxford Textbook of Medical Education. Oxford University Press, Oxford (Chapter 33).

35

Curriculum evaluation is an essential part of the educational process. The focus in curriculum evaluation is on quality improvement.

Why evaluate the curriculum?

The earlier chapters in this section are concerned with the evaluation of the student. In this chapter we look at the evaluation of the curriculum of a medical school or educational organisation. Curriculum evaluation can be defined as 'a deliberate act of enquiry which sets out with the intention of allowing people concerned with an educational event to make rigorous, informed judgements and decisions about it so that appropriate development may be facilitated' (Coles and Grant 1985).

The education programme as described in earlier chapters is complex, involving multiple interactions. Evaluation therefore is not easy. The evaluation can be conducted at the level of medical school, the curriculum, a course in the curriculum, e.g. 'an introduction to clinical medicine', a subject, e.g. the behavioural sciences, or a learning event such as a lecture or clinical teaching session.

The evaluation of a curriculum can have different purposes. It can be used to:

- Demonstrate that the curriculum is fit for purpose as determined by the achievement of the minimum standards expected by an accrediting body such as the General Medical Council in the UK, the Liaison Committee on Medical Education (LCME) in the United States or the Australian Medical Council (AMC) in Australia. The World Federation for Medical Education (WFME) has set out minimum standards for educational programmes at undergraduate, postgraduate and continuing education levels. An ongoing evaluation approach linked to accreditation standards is valuable (Barzansky et al. 2015).
- Establish that the programme as set out on paper ('the intended or planned curriculum') corresponds with the curriculum in action ('the taught or received curriculum') and what the student learns ('the learned curriculum'). There is often a gap between what is set out on paper and what happens in practice.

- Identify the strengths and weaknesses of the curriculum, as part of an internal iterative process, with feedback provided where problems are identified and where change is required.
- Inform curriculum development. Without an evaluation of the curriculum there can be no informed curriculum change. Curriculum evaluation should be concerned not simply with a measurement of the success or failure of a curricular initiative but should be a more complex assessment that provides a fuller understanding of the education process. Parlett and Hamilton (1975) describe this as 'illuminative evaluation'.
- Assess curriculum change. A better understanding of a change made to the curriculum can be sought and the extent to which it has been effective measured. The difference between curriculum evaluation and research is sometimes questioned. As argued by Kelly (2004), curriculum evaluation becomes part of curriculum research. In the context of research, the findings of the evaluation must be examined from a generalisable perspective. Curriculum planning and evaluation can be seen as a hypothesis to be tested.
- Compare education programmes in institutions in different countries or an institution with different approaches and admission policies. Such information is useful in the context of student mobility as well as for use in research in medical education.
- Meet specific needs of stakeholders. The government may be interested, for example, in the number of students graduating who choose primary care as a career, and choose to work in rural areas or the number who become the academics of the future.
- Provide information for a wider audience, including potential students, as to areas of excellence in the education programme in a medical school as judged, for example, by the ASPIRE-to-excellence criteria (see Chapter 21). The publication by the Higher Education Funding Councils in the UK of the ratings of the education programmes in medical schools was associated with significant changes in the pattern of schools to which students applied to be admitted.

Focus for the evaluation

An evaluation of the education programme can be conceptualised at different levels:

- At the *macro* level the mission of the medical school and the extent to which the school is achieving its overall aims can be examined.
- At the *micro* level the elements of the curriculum can be evaluated. These include the learning outcomes, the teaching, learning and assessment methods, the educational strategies, the education environment, the management of the curriculum and the engagement with students and staff.

The CIPP approach

CIPP refers to context, input, process and product, the four elements addressed in an evaluation:

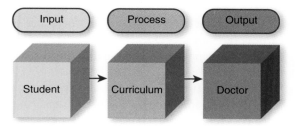

Figure 35.1 Evaluation of the input, the process and the output

- the *context* in which the school is operating and the needs it is expected to meet
- the *input* in terms of students enrolled and the resources provided
- the *process* through which the education programme is delivered
- the *product* or doctors produced.

Value-added assessment

In value-added-assessment an evaluation of the quality of the product or the students graduating from a school takes into account the students admitted to medical studies. This is important, particularly where a policy has been implemented of broadening access to medical studies so that the doctors qualified better reflect the population they are to serve. How does the school cope with the less able and the more able students? To what extent does the school smooth the pebbles as well as polish the diamonds?

The 'ten questions' framework for curriculum evaluation

The ten questions to be addressed in the planning of a curriculum, as described in Chapter 13, can be used also as a framework for a curriculum evaluation. Examples are given of the issues to be addressed relating to each question.

1. **The needs the medical school aims to meet**
   - Is the mission of the medical school stated and communicated to all the stakeholders?
   - Does the mission of the school reflect its social responsibility?
   - Some schools see as their mission the development of future leaders or researchers. Others see their mission in terms of the social responsibility and accountability of the school and how it relates to the community that it serves. Boelen and Woollard (2009) have argued that for a school to be socially responsible it needs to have a commitment to respond to the priority health needs of citizens and society. The impact of the educational institution on society and the public good should be part of the assessment of its success. It has been shown that the most research-active medical schools demonstrate the least social responsibility.

2. **Learning outcomes**
   - Is there a clear statement shared with the teachers and students about the expected learning outcomes?
   - Have the stakeholders, including patients and those concerned with other phases of education, had an input to this?
   - Are decisions about the curriculum based on these learning outcomes? A framework to assess the implementation of outcome-based education in a medical school is described in Chapter 10.
   - Is the school equipping its graduates as citizens of the world with a sound knowledge of global issues, the skills for working in an international context and the values of a global citizen?

3. **The curriculum content**
   - What content is addressed in the curriculum and how does this relate to the stated learning outcomes? How are new subjects such as genetics addressed alongside more traditional subjects?
   - Has a core curriculum been defined with threshold concepts?
   - How is the danger of information overload addressed?

4. **Sequence and organisation**
   - What consideration has been given to the organisation and sequencing of content within the curriculum?
   - To what extent is there exposure to clinical experiences early in the programme and to the basic medical sciences later?

5. **Educational strategies**

The 'SPICES' model as described in Chapter 13 is a useful tool to analyse the curriculum and the educational strategies:

   - Student-centred/Teacher-centred
   - Problem-based/Information-based
   - Integrated/Discipline-based
   - Community-orientated/Hospital-orientated
   - Electives/Uniform
   - Systematic/Opportunistic

Where is the school placed on each continuum between the two extremes?

6. **Teaching and learning methods and opportunities**
   - To what extent have new approaches to teaching and learning such as simulation and e-learning been adopted?
   - Have these approaches been adapted to meet local needs?
   - Is there a grid or blueprint that relates the expected learning outcomes to the available learning opportunities?
   - To what extent has there been a move to more 'authentic learning'?
   - To what extent is collaborative or peer-to-peer learning encouraged and developed?
   - To what extent are the international dimensions to learning incorporated?

- What use is made of lectures?
- To what extent is there engagement with the students as partners in the learning process, including peer teaching?

7. **Assessment**
   - To what extent is assessment blueprinted against the learning outcomes?
   - To what extent is the rich range of tools now available harnessed to assess students' competence?
   - Is there a measure of the students' progression through the curriculum?
   - Is there adequate feedback to the students and teachers?

8. **Educational environment**
   - How can the education environment in the medical school be characterised and is this in line with the expected learning outcomes?
   - Has the education environment been measured using a tool as described in Chapter 21?

9. **Communication about the curriculum**
   - How is the information about the medical curriculum communicated to staff, students and other stakeholders?
   - Is a discussion about the curriculum on the agenda for Faculty Board meetings?
   - Is there a curriculum planning committee with responsibility for the curriculum?
   - Is a curriculum map available?

10. **Management**
    - Who makes decisions about the curriculum and does the management structure support the implementation of the curriculum?
    - Are the roles of the teachers defined and matched to their abilities?
    - How is teaching recognised and rewarded within the medical school?
    - Is a staff development programme implemented?
    - How are teachers kept up to date with advances in medical education and in their own specialty?
    - What sort of quality assurance processes are in place?
    - Are plans in place for the ongoing and further development of the curriculum?

Kirkpatrick's four levels of evaluation

Kirkpatrick described four levels for assessing the effectiveness of training. Although the model was developed for use in a business context it has been widely applied in medical education. Each successive level in the model provides a more precise measure of the effectiveness of the educational programme but requires a more rigorous and time-consuming analysis. Evaluation can begin at the first level and, as time and resources allow, move to the higher levels (Figure 35.2).

Level 1: Opinion/reaction. Evaluation at this level examines how participants in the education programme react to it. Are they satisfied? Do they like or dislike it? Does it meet their needs?

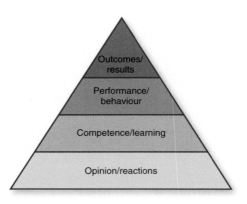

Figure 35.2 Kirkpatrick's four levels

Level 2: Competence/learning. This level moves beyond the learner's satisfaction. The extent to which there is a difference in the learner's knowledge, skills or attitudes is assessed. Students' performance in written or clinical assessments is studied and taken as evidence of the effectiveness of the education programme.

Level 3: Performance/behaviour transfer. Changes in the learner's behaviour are studied at this level. As a result of the education programme do students communicate more effectively in their day-to-day contacts with patients? Do students apply their knowledge of the basic sciences to understand better the pathophysiology of patients they encounter?

Level 4: Outcome/results. This level, in the context of Kirkpatrick's work, measures the success of a training programme in terms of the business results. Did sales increase after training was completed? In medical education the question is whether the training of the doctor affects medical practice. Does the training in cardiac auscultation and the interpretation of murmurs, for example, reduce the need for laboratory investigations of patients? Does education of doctors about hypertension reduce the incidence of side effects in patients presenting with raised blood pressure?

Undertaking a curriculum evaluation

Undertaking a curriculum evaluation involves:

- Clarifying the purpose of the evaluation. A number of different aims are mentioned earlier in the chapter.
- Deciding the approach to be adopted. The CIPP approach, the 'ten questions' model and the Kirkpatrick 'four levels' approach are described.
- Deciding the evidence to be collected. This may include:
  - the curriculum outline, including details of the core and optional elements of the course
  - the statement of the expected learning outcomes
  - the timetable and schedule for individual students

- the curriculum management structure and responsibility for decisions
- results of assessment of student performance
- students' perceptions of the curriculum
- teachers' perceptions of the curriculum
- follow-up of graduates, including their views on the curriculum, their career, their achievement and problems encountered in practice and disciplinary action.
- Engaging the stakeholders. These include the curriculum committee, the teachers, the students, other health professionals, future employers and the public.
- Planning the methods to be used. These almost certainly will include qualitative and quantitative methods.
- Allocating responsibilities for the implementation of the evaluation and the necessary resources to carry it out.
- Planning how the results will be communicated and how action will be taken as a result of the evaluation.

Over to you

Reflect and react

1. Are you aware of the stated mission for your medical school or educational body? How successfully is this achieved?
2. Which of the purposes described for curriculum evaluation are relevant to your situation?
3. What steps are taken to evaluate your curriculum and are all the stakeholders involved? Is effective use made of the results of the evaluation?

Explore further

Journal articles

Barzansky, B., Hunt, D., Moineau, G., et al., 2015. Continuous quality improvement in an accreditation system for undergraduate medical education: benefits and challenges. Med. Teach. 37 (11), 1032–1038.
Links ongoing curriculum evaluation to accreditation standards.
Boelen, C., Woollard, B., 2009. Social accountability and accreditation: a new frontier for educational institutions. Med. Educ. 43, 887–894.
An account of social accountability as a mission of a medical school.
Coles, C.R., Grant, J.G., 1985. Curriculum evaluation in medical and healthcare education. Med. Educ. 19, 405–442.
A description of what is meant by curriculum evaluation in medical education.

Harden, R.M., 1986. Ten questions to ask when planning a course or curriculum. Med. Educ. 20, 356–365.
A description of the ten questions to be asked when planning a curriculum.

Guides

Frye, A.W., Hemmer, P.A., 2012. Program evaluation models and related theories. AMEE Guide No. 67. Med. Teach. 34, 288–299.
A review of the theoretical basics for models for curriculum evaluation to assist the teacher in their role as a curriculum evaluator.
Goldie, J., 2006. Evaluating educational programmes. AMEE Education Guide No. 29. Med. Teach. 28, 210–224.
Practical advice on curriculum evaluation.

Books

Berk, R.A., 2006. Thirteen Strategies to Measure College Teaching. A Consumer's Guide to Rating Scale Construction, Assessment, and Decision Making for Faculty, Administrators, and Clinicians. Stylus Publishing, Virginia.

An amusingly written account of how to assess the effectiveness of teaching.

Kelly, A.V., 2004. The Curriculum: Theory and Practice, 5th ed. Sage, London.

A useful account of the purpose, approaches and theory underpinning curriculum evaluation.

Kirkpatrick, D., Kirkpatrick, J., 2006. Evaluating Training Programs: The Four Levels, third ed. Berrett-Koehler, San Francisco.

Parlett, M., Hamilton, D., 1975. Evaluation as illumination. In: Tawney, D. (Ed.), Curriculum Evaluation Today: Trends and Implications. Schools Council Research Studies. Macmillan, London.

A classic description of illuminative education.

Websites

World Federation for Medical Education (WFME). <http://wfme.org/standards>.

APPENDICES

1. Entrustable Professional Activities (EPAs) for undergraduate medical education as specified by the Association of American Medical Colleges (AAMC)   268
2. The learning outcomes for a competent practitioner based on the three-circle model   269
3. Four dimensions of student progression   271
4. A page from a study guide, 'Learning paediatrics: a training guide for senior house officers'   272
5. Summary of various points in the continuum between a problem-based approach and an information-oriented approach   273
6. The clinical presentations that provide a framework for the curriculum in task-based learning   275
7. First two sections of the learning outcome/tasks mastery grid for vocational training in dentistry   277
8. Dundee Ready Education Environment Measure (DREEM)   278
9. Examples of OSCE stations   279

APPENDIX 1

ENTRUSTABLE PROFESSIONAL ACTIVITIES (EPAS) FOR UNDERGRADU-ATE MEDICAL EDUCATION AS SPECIFIED BY THE ASSOCIATION OF AMERICAN MEDICAL COLLEGES (AAMC) (Greenberg, R., 2014. Core Entrustable Professional Activities for entering residency. https://www.aamc.org/cepaer)

1. Gather a history and perform a physical examination
2. Prioritise a differential diagnosis following a clinical encounter
3. Recommend and interpret common diagnostic and screening tests
4. Enter and discuss orders and prescriptions
5. Document a clinical encounter in the patient record
6. Provide an oral presentation of a clinical encounter
7. Form clinical questions and retrieve evidence to advance patient care
8. Give or receive a patient handover to transition care responsibility
9. Collaborate as a member of an interprofessional team
10. Recognise a patient requiring urgent or emergent care and initiate evaluation and management
11. Obtain informed consent for tests and/or procedures
12. Perform general procedures of a physician
13. Identify system failures and contribute to a culture of safety and improvement

APPENDIX 2

THE LEARNING OUTCOMES FOR A COMPETENT PRACTITIONER BASED ON THE THREE-CIRCLE MODEL (reproduced with permission from Harden et al., 1999. AMEE Guide No. 14: Outcome-based education Part 5)

A						
What the doctor is able to do – 'doing the right thing'						
Technical Intelligences						
Clinical skills	Practical procedures	Patient investigation	Patient management	Health promotion and disease prevention	Communication	Appropriate information handling skills
History Physical examination Interpretation of findings Formulation of action plan	Cardiology Dermatology Endocrinology Gastroenterology Haematology Musculo skeletal Nervous system Ophthalmology Otolaryngology	General principles Clinical imaging Biochemical medicine Haematology Immunology	General principles Drugs Surgery Psychological Physiotherapy Radiotherapy Social Nutrition Emergency medicine Acute care	Recognition of causes of threats to health and individuals at risk Implementation where appropriate of basics of prevention Collaboration with other health professionals in health promotion and disease prevention	With patient With relatives With colleagues With media/ press Teaching Managing Patient advocate Mediation and negotiation By telephone In writing	Patient records Accessing data sources Use of computers Implementation of professional guidelines Personal records (log books, portfolios)

B			C	
How the doctor approaches their practice – 'doing the thing right'			**The doctor as a professional – 'the right person doing it'**	
Intellectual Intelligences	*Emotional Intelligences*	*Analytical and creative Intelligences*	*Personal Intelligences*	
Understanding of social, basic and clinical sciences and underlying principles	Appropriate attitudes, ethical understanding and legal responsibilities	Appropriate decision making skills, and clinical reasoning and judgement	Role of the doctor within the health service	Personal development
Normal structure and function	Attitudes	Clinical reasoning	Understanding of healthcare systems	Self learner
Normal behaviour	Understanding of ethical principles	Evidence-based medicine	Understanding of clinical responsibilities and role of doctor	Self awareness
The life cycle	Ethical standards	Critical thinking		Enquires into own competence
Pathophysiology	Legal responsibilities	Research method		
Psychosocial model of illness	Human rights issues	Statistical understanding	Acceptance of code of conduct and required personal attributes	Emotional awareness
Pharmacology and clinical pharmacology	Respect for colleagues	Creativity/ resourcefulness	Appreciation of doctor as researcher	Self confidence
	Medicine in multicultural societies	Coping with uncertainty	Appreciation of doctor as mentor or teacher	Self regulation
Public health medicine	Awareness of psychosocial issues	Prioritisation	Appreciation of doctor as manager including quality control	Self care
Epidemiology	Awareness of economic issues			Self control
Preventative medicine and health prevention	Acceptance of responsibility to contribute to advance of medicine		Appreciation of doctor as member of multi-professional team and of roles of other healthcare professionals	Adaptability to change
Education	Appropriate attitude to professional institution and health service bodies			Personal time management
Health economics				Motivation
				Achievement drive
				Commitment
				Initiative
				Career choice

APPENDIX 3

FOUR DIMENSIONS OF STUDENT PROGRESSION (reproduced with permission from Harden, R.M., 2007. Learning outcomes as a tool to assess progression. Med. Teach. 29, 678-682)

Increased scope

Increased Breadth	*Increased Difficulty*
A → A + B + C	A → A

• Extension to more or new topics
• Extension to different practice contexts
• Application of existing knowledge or skills to new knowledge or skills
	• More in-depth or advances consideration
	• Application to a more complex situation
	  • move from a uni-dimensional straightforward situation to one involving multiple problems or systems
	  • move to multifactorial problems involving different factors (e.g. social, economical, medical)
	  • complications (e.g. associated with treatment)
	• Less obvious or more subtle situations
	  • fewer cues
	  • less obvious cues
	  • atypical cues

Increased utility

Application (to medical practice)

A → A

Increased proficiency

Increased Accomplishment

A → A

• Move from general context to specific medical context
• Move from theory to practice of medicine
• Move to integration into the role of a doctor
  • an integrated repertoire involving a holistic approach to practice and bringing together the different abilities expected of a doctor
  • dealing with and reconciling competing demands, such as time spent on curative and preventive medicine
	• More efficient performance
	  • better organised
	  • more confident
	  • takes less time
	  • more accessible
	  • less unnecessary or redundant action
	  • higher standards
	  • lower errors
	• Less need for supervision
	• Takes initiative and anticipates events
	• Better able to defend and justify actions
	• Adapts routinely as part of practice

APPENDIX 4

A PAGE FROM A STUDY GUIDE, 'LEARNING PAEDIATRICS: A TRAINING GUIDE FOR SENIOR HOUSE OFFICERS' (reproduced with permission from Harden, R.M., Laidlaw, J.M., Hesketh, E.A., 1999. Study guides – their use and preparation. AMEE Medical Education Guide No. 16. Med. Teach. 21, 248-265)

Therapy

Strict schedules governing oral intake are not helpful. Discuss with nursing and medical staff when oral fluids or diet should be increased or reintroduced.

Black's *Paediatric Emergencies* has several useful sections.
• Appendix 3, p766-769 (water and electrolyte requirements)
• Appendix 5, p773-755 (advice on necessary maintenance fluids)

For an overview of home-based oral rehydration for diarrhoea, Almroth & Lathham, *Lancet*, Mar 1995; 345(8951) 709-711.

A Meyes, Modern management of acute diarrhoea and dehydration in children. *Am Fam Phys*, Apr 1995: 57(5): 1103-1118, may also give you some ideas.

Teamwork

Speak to colleagues in the local Public Health Department. Discuss infection-control policies and notification of diseases.

Experienced nursing staff may help you decide on the best method of rehydration. Remember – you can always reassess cases after a few hours and review your decisions.

Professional development

Do you know how to prevent cross contamination?

With each case, consider what measures may be required e.g. hand washing alone, or additional gloves, masks and gowns.

Think why a child is being barrier nursed. Is it to protect the patient or the staff/other patients/environment?

Look at the local infection-control policy for guidance.

Microbiology in Clinical Practice (p602-607) contains a short section on different standards of isolation, with suggested isolation procedures.

APPENDIX 5

SUMMARY OF VARIOUS POINTS IN THE CONTINUUM BETWEEN A PROBLEM-BASED APPROACH AND AN INFORMATION-ORIENTED APPROACH

'Rul' is the rules or principles to be learned. 'Eg' is the problem or clinical example addressed by the student. (Reproduced with permission. First published in Harden, R.M., Davis, M.H., 1998. The continuum of problem-based learning. Med. Teach. 20, 317-322)

	Terminology	Description	Example
1	Theoretical learning.	Information provided about the theory.	Traditional lecture. Standard textbook.
2	Problem-orientated learning.	Practical information provided.	Lecture with practical information. Protocols or guidelines.
3	Problem-assisted learning.	Information provided with the opportunity to apply it to practical examples.	Lecture followed by practical or clinical experience. Book with problems or experiences included.
4	Problem-solving learning.	Problem-solving related to specific examples.	Case discussions and some activities in practical classes.
5	Problem-focused learning.	Information is provided followed by a problem. The principles of the subject are then learned.	Introductory or foundation courses or lecture. Information in study guide.
6	Problem-based mixed approach.	A combination of problem-based and information-based learning.	Students have the option of an information-orientated or problem-based approach.
7	Problem-initiated learning.	The problem is used as a trigger at the beginning of learning.	Patient management problems are used to interest the student in a topic.

	Terminology	Description	Example
8 Eg → Rul(Sp)	Problem-centred learning.	A study of the problem introduces the student to the principles and rules specific to the problem.	A text provides a series of problems followed by the information necessary to tackle the problems.
9 Eg ⇢ Rul(Sp)	Problem-centred discovery learning.	Following the presentation of the problem students have the opportunity to derive the principles and rules.	Students derive the principles from the literature or from work undertaken.
10 Eg → Rul(G)	Problem-based learning.	The development of the principles includes the generalisation stage of learning.	The investigation of patients with thyrotoxicosis is extended to a more general understanding of thyroid function tests.
11 Eg(T) → Rul	Task-based learning.	The problem is the real world.	A set of tasks undertaken by a health care professional are the basis for the 'problem' presented to the student.

APPENDIX 6

THE CLINICAL PRESENTATIONS THAT PROVIDE A FRAMEWORK FOR THE CURRICULUM IN TASK-BASED LEARNING (reproduced with permission from Harden, R.M., Crosby, J.R., Davis, M.H., et al., 2000. Task-based learning: the answer to integration and problem-based learning in the clinical years. Med. Educ. 34, 391-397)

1. **Pain**
   Pain in the leg on walking
   Acute abdominal pain
   Loin pain and dysuria
   Joint pain
   Back and neck pain
   Indigestion
   Headache
   Cancer pain
   Earache
2. **Bleeding and bruising**
   Bruising easily
   Pallor
   Haemoptysis
   Vomiting blood
   Rectal bleeding
   Blood in urine
   Anaemia
   Post-operative bleeding
3. **Fever and infection**
   Chest infection
   Rash and fever
   Urethral discharge
   Pyrexia of unknown origin
   Immunisation
   Sweating
   Hypothermia
   Sepsis
4. **Altered consciousness**
   Immobility
   Falls
   Collapse
   Confusion
   Dizziness
   Fits
5. **Paralysis and impaired mobility**
   Loss of power on one side
   Tremor

Peripheral neuropathy
Muscle weakness
Immobility
Falling over
6. **Lumps, bumps and swelling**
   Lump in the neck
   Lump in groin
   Lump in breast
   Swollen scrotum
   Joint swelling
   Swollen ankles
   Skin lump
7. **Nutrition/weight**
   Thirsty and losing weight
   Difficulty swallowing
   Weight loss
   Seriously overweight
8. **Change in body function**
   Wheezing
   Pleural effusion
   Shortness of breath
   Cough
   Change in bowel habit
   Cannot pass urine
   Incontinence
   Raised blood pressure
   Palpitations
9. **Skin problems**
   Skin rash
   Itching
   Psoriasis
   Mole growing bigger/bleeding
   Blistering
   Photosensitivity
   Bedsore
   Jaundice
   Burn
   Wound

10. **Life threatening/Accident and Emergency**
    Shock
    Involvement in accident
    Fracture
11. **Eyes**
    Loss of vision
    Painful red eyes
    Squinting in child
    Foreign body in child
12. **Ear, nose and throat**
    Ringing in ear
    Going deaf
    Earache
    Sore throat
    Hoarseness
    Stuffy nose
13. **Behaviour**
    Anger
    Anxiety
    Phobias
    Drug addiction
    Suicide
    Sleep problems
    Bereavement
    Alcohol dependence
    Schizophrenia
    Tiredness
    Depression
    Adolescence
14. **Reproductive problems**
    Pre-menstrual syndrome
    Infertility
    Normal pregnancy
    Menstrual problems
    Contraception
    Sterilisation
    Smear results
    Painful intercourse
15. **The child**
    Child abuse
    Down syndrome
    Prematurity
    Poor feeding
    Failure to thrive
    Respiratory distress syndrome
    Developmental delay
    Sudden infant death syndrome/
        near miss
16. **Priority setting, decision making and audit**
    Dying patient
    Population screening
    Waiting lists
    Triage
    Acute vs chronic

APPENDIX 7

FIRST TWO SECTIONS OF THE LEARNING OUTCOME/TASKS MASTERY GRID FOR VOCATIONAL TRAINING IN DENTISTRY (reproduced from Mitchell, H.E., Harden, R.M., Laidlaw, I.M., 1999. Med. Teach. 20, 91–98)

	Tasks performed by the trainee*					
	Caries and restorations	Periodontal patient	Acute dental pain	Endodontic problem	Partial/complete denture	Minor surgical procedure
General						
Critically appraise and assess his or her own work	+	+	+	+	+	+
Keep up to date and continue with his or her education	+	+	+	+	+	+
Understand not only what he or she is doing, but why it is being done	+	+	+	+	+	+
Communication with patients						
History taking	+	+	+	+	+	+
Explanation of the clinical condition	+	+	+	+	+	+
Explanation of suggested treatment plan and alternatives	+	+	+	+	+	+
Explanation of cost and obtaining consent to pay	+	±	±	+	+	+
Explanation of preventive aspects of the patient's problem	+	+	+	+	–	+
Explanation of recognised complications related to treatment	+	–	+	+	+	–
Explanation of appliance inconvenience or failure	–	–	–	–	+	–
Explanation of necessary appliance	–	–	–	–	+	–

*applies +; may apply ±; does not apply –.

APPENIDX 8

DUNDEE READY EDUCATION ENVIRONMENT MEASURE (DREEM)
(reproduced with permission from McAleer, S., Roff, S., 2001. Curriculum, Climate, Quality and Change in Medical Education: A Unifying Perspective. AMEE Guide No. 23. Part 3 Appendix 1)

Dundee Ready Education Measure (DREEM)

Age [ ]   Year of study [ ]   Male [ ]   Female [ ]

Medical School [ ]

Please indicate whether you:
Strongly Agree (SA), Agree (A), are Unsure (U), Disagree (D) or Strongly Disagree (SD) with the following statements. Circle the appropriate response.

	SA	A	U	D	SD
1. I am encouraged to participate in class	SA	A	U	D	SD
2. The teachers are knowledgeable	SA	A	U	D	SD
3. There is a good support system for students who get stressed	SA	A	U	D	SD
4. I am too tired to enjoy the course	SA	A	U	D	SD
5. Learning strategies which worked for me before continue to work for me now	SA	A	U	D	SD
6. The teachers are patient with patients	SA	A	U	D	SD
7. The teaching is often stimulating	SA	A	U	D	SD
8. The teachers ridicule the students	SA	A	U	D	SD
9. The teachers are authoritarian	SA	A	U	D	SD
10. I am confident about my passing this year	SA	A	U	D	SD
11. The atmosphere is relaxed during the ward teaching	SA	A	U	D	SD
12. The school is well time tabled	SA	A	U	D	SD
13. The teaching is student centred	SA	A	U	D	SD
14. I am rarely bored on this course	SA	A	U	D	SD
15. I have good friends in this school	SA	A	U	D	SD
16. The teaching helps to develop my competence	SA	A	U	D	SD
17. Cheating is a problem in this school	SA	A	U	D	SD
18. The teachers have good communication skills with patients	SA	A	U	D	SD
19. My social life is good	SA	A	U	D	SD
20. The teaching is well focused	SA	A	U	D	SD
21. I feel I am being well prepared for my profession	SA	A	U	D	SD
22. The teaching helps to develop my confidence	SA	A	U	D	SD
23. The atmosphere is relaxed during lectures	SA	A	U	D	SD
24. The teaching time is put to good use	SA	A	U	D	SD
25. The teaching over-emphasises factual learning	SA	A	U	D	SD
26. Last year's work has been a good preparation for this year's work	SA	A	U	D	SD
27. I am able to memorise all I need	SA	A	U	D	SD
28. I seldom feel lonely	SA	A	U	D	SD
29. The teachers are good at providing feedback to students	SA	A	U	D	SD
30. There are opportunities for me to develop interpersonal skills	SA	A	U	D	SD
31. I have learned a lot about empathy in my profession	SA	A	U	D	SD
32. The teachers provide constructive criticism here	SA	A	U	D	SD
33. I feel comfortable in class socially	SA	A	U	D	SD
34. The atmosphere is relaxed during seminars/tutorials	SA	A	U	D	SD
35. I find the experience disappointing	SA	A	U	D	SD
36. I am able to concentrate well	SA	A	U	D	SD
37. The teachers give clear examples	SA	A	U	D	SD
38. I am clear about the learning objectives of the course	SA	A	U	D	SD
39. The teachers get angry in class	SA	A	U	D	SD
40. The teachers are well prepared for their classes	SA	A	U	D	SD
41. My problem solving skills are being well developed here	SA	A	U	D	SD
42. The enjoyment outweighs the stress of the course	SA	A	U	D	SD
43. The atmosphere motivates me as a learner	SA	A	U	D	SD
44. The teaching encourages me to be an active learner	SA	A	U	D	SD
45. Much of what I have to learn seems relevant to a career in healthcare	SA	A	U	D	SD
46. My accommodation is pleasant	SA	A	U	D	SD
47. Long term learning is emphasised over short term learning	SA	A	U	D	SD
48. The teaching to too teacher-centred	SA	A	U	D	SD
49. I feel able to ask the questions I want	SA	A	U	D	SD
50. The students irritate the teachers	SA	A	U	D	SD

APPENDIX 9

EXAMPLES OF OSCE STATIONS

- History taking from a patient who presents with a problem, e.g. abdominal pain.
- History taking to elucidate a diagnosis, e.g. hypothyroidism.
- Educating a patient about management, e.g. use of inhaler for asthma.
- Advice to a patient and his wife, e.g. on discharge from hospital with a myocardial infarction.
- Explanation to a patient about tests and procedures, e.g. endoscopy.
- Communication with other members of healthcare teams, e.g. brief to nurse with regard to a terminally ill patient.
- Communication with relatives, e.g. informing a wife that her husband has bronchial carcinoma.
- Physical examination of system or part of body, e.g. examination of hands.
- Physical examination to follow up a problem identified, e.g. congestive cardiac failure.
- Physical examination to help confirm or refute a diagnosis, e.g. thyrotoxicosis.
- A diagnostic procedure, e.g. ophthalmoscopy.
- Written communication, e.g. writing referral letter or discharge letter.
- Interpretation of findings and follow-up action, e.g. charts, laboratory reports or findings documented in patient's records.
- Management, e.g. writing a prescription or commentary on a prescription.
- Critical appraisal, e.g. review of published article or pharmaceutical advertisement.
- Management of errors, e.g. meet with a senior hospital administrator to follow up a letter of complaint from a patient who complains that her weight as recorded was not her correct weight and initiate the action to be taken.

Index

Page numbers followed by "*f*" indicate figures, "*b*" indicate boxes, and "*t*" indicate tables.

A

A European Union High Level Group: Train the professors to teach, 4
Academic record, 255
Accountability, outcome-based education and, 59–60
Accreditation Council for Graduate Medical Education (ACGME), 75–76
Accrediting bodies, value of curriculum mapping to, 161
Accrediting Committee for Graduate Medical Education (ACGME), 67
Action-based learning, 133
Active learning, 18–19
Activity, students learning through, 15, 18–20
Adaptive learning, 112–113
development of, 22
Administrators, value of curriculum mapping to, 161
Advances in Health Sciences Education and Academic Medicine, 52
The Aims of Education, 27
Altered consciousness, 275
Ambulatory care, 197
Anaesthetic theatre educational environment measure (ATEEM), 157
Anatomical Sciences Education, 52
Apprenticeship, 99, 135–143
see also Work-based learning
Apprenticeship model, 135
Aptitude tests, 256
Assessment, 217, 219–229
of curriculum. *see* Curriculum, evaluation
of education environment, 156–157
importance of, 219–220
of students. *see* Student assessment
written and computer-based, 231–236, 232*f*

elements in, 231–233
role of, 231
technology, 235–236
types of, 233–235
Assessors, teachers as, 9–10, 219
in e-learning, 205
Association for Medical Education in Europe (AMEE), 35, 52
Association of American Medical Colleges (AAMC), Entrustable Professional Activities (EPAS) for undergraduate medical education as specified by, 268
Attitudes
development of, in students, 223
to teaching, 12
Audience, engaging, 170
'Authentic academic tasks', 90–91
'Authentic' curriculum, 89–94
features of, 91
from university to real world, 89–94, 91*f*
Autobiographical narrative, 255
Awareness, integration continuum, 127

B

Beavers, outcome-based education implementation, 81
Behaviour, 276
Best Evidence Medical Education (BEME) Collaboration, 35, 37, 37*f*
Bleeding and bruising, 275
Blended learning, 206–207
Body systems, integrated learning of, 127
Boyer, E.L., 12–13
Brainstorming, 177
Breadth, increased, in student progression, 271*f*
Bridging programme, 106
British Education Index (BEI), 35–36

Brown abilities, 76–77
Burn out, 30–31

C

CanMEDS physician competency framework, 75, 76*f*
Case-based discussion (CbD), 241
Centre for the Advancement of Interprofessional Education (CAIPE), 131–132
Child, 276
Classroom, flipped, 171–174
advantages and disadvantages of, 172–173
comparison of the traditional lecture and, 172*f*
definition of, 171–172
implementation in practice, 173–174
medical education, application in, 172
Climate, educational, 100–101
Clinical and performance-based assessment, 237–245
approaches to, 239–242
the examiner in, 242–243
importance of, 237
the patient in, 237–239
portfolio, 242
Clinical context, teaching and learning in, 189–194
Clinical experience, early, 104
Clinical setting
task-based learning in, 120
see also Clinical teaching
Clinical skills centres, 200–202
Clinical supervision, 193–194
Clinical teaching
changing perceptions of, 189–190, 189*f*, 191*t*
clinical supervision in, 193–194
implementing, 192–193
planning, 192–193

Clinical teaching (Continued)
  postgraduate training, 190
  role of patient in, 191–192
  role of student in, 190
  role of teacher in, 190, 191t
  in small groups, 178
  teaching procedural skills in, 192
  student progression, 192
Collaboration
  between different phases of
    medical education, 42–44, 43f
  importance of, 41
  with other health care
    professionals, 44
  with other stakeholders, 44
  with others within your institution,
    42
  in practice, 45–47
  between teachers
    within medical school, 42
    with the responsibility for a
      similar programme locally,
      nationally or internationally,
      44–45, 45f
Collaboration: What Makes It Work,
  45–46
Collaborative learning, 211–216
  benefits of, 212–213
  definition of, 211–212
  examples of, 212
  implementation in practice,
    214–216
Collaborative orientation, in
  education environment, 155
Colleagues
  evidence from, 35
  feedback from, 18, 51
Communities of practice, keeping up
  to date from, 52–53
Community orientation, in education
  environment, 155–156
Community-based education,
  136–137
  definition of, 136
  rationale for, 136
  urban and rural setting, 136–137
Community-based learning, 98
  implementation of, 137
  see also Work-based learning
Competencies
  assessment of, 237
  in clinical and performance-based
    assessment, 242
  communicating, 73–79
  describing, 73–79
  enquiring into your own, 50–51
  and Entrustable Professional
    Activities, 63–64, 63f
  gained, application of, 104
  of good teacher, 10f, 11
  and outcome-based education, 57,
    59
  and portfolio assessment, 249
  specification of, 67–71

Competency-based approach, move
  to, 57–65
Competency-based education (CBE),
  57
  definition of, 58–59, 58f
Competency-based student
  assessment, 224
Competitive orientation, in education
  environment, 155
Complementary programme,
  integration continuum, 129
Computer(s)
  in e-learning, 203
  simulations, 239
Conferences, keeping up to date
  from, 52
Consortium of Longitudinal
  Integrated Clerkships (CLIC), 138
Context, input, process and product
  (CIPP) approach, 260–261, 261f
Contextualised learning, 208
Continuity, outcome-based
  education and, 60
Continuum of education, 43f
  curriculum mapping in, 160
Cookbook approach, 15
Cooperative learning, 208
Core curriculum
  advantages of, with SSCs, 146–147,
    147f
  responding to information
    overload and building options
    into, 145–151
  specification of, 147–148
Correlation, integration continuum,
  129
Course content, 103
Courses, on medical education,
  keeping up to date from, 52
Creative Collaboration, 46–47
CRISIS framework, 205, 205f
Criterion-referenced approach to
  student assessment, 221
Critical incident survey, 69–70
Cumulative Index to Nursing and
  Allied Health Literature (CINAHL),
  35–36
Curriculum, 3–4, 3f, 89
  actual, 92
  adaptive elements into, 22–23
  'authentic', 89–94
  features of, 91
  from university to real world,
    89–94, 91f
  communication of details of, 100
  concept of, 89
  content of, 96–97
  organised, 97
  core
    advantages of, with SSCs,
      146–147, 147f
    responding to information
      overload and building options
      into, 145–151

specification of, 147–148
delivered, 92–94, 93f
development, 87
educational environment or
  climate, 100–101
educational strategies for, 97–99,
  97f
Entrustable Professional Activities
  and, 64–65
evaluation, 259–266
  aims of, 260
  approaches to, 260
  curriculum mapping in, 160
  definition of, 259
  focus for, 260–261
  illuminative, 260
  Kirkpatrick's four levels of,
    263–264, 264f
  ten questions framework,
    261–263
  undertaking, 264–266
  value-added assessment, 261
expected learning outcomes, 96
hidden, 92–94
integration, simulators and, 199
learned, 92–94, 93f
mapping, 159–163
  definition of, 159
  need for, 159
  potential users of, 160–161,
    161f
  preparing, 162–163
  outcome-based education,
  student progression in, 82
planned, 92–94, 93f, 259
planners
  in e-learning, teachers as, 206
  teachers as, 9–10
  value of curriculum mapping to,
    161
planning
  in problem-based learning, 119
  questions to ask when, 95–101
  trends in, 135
  problems in, outcome-based
    education and, 60
  progression, 106
  received, 259
  role of independent learning in,
    184–185
  sequencing content of, 103–106
  basic and clinical sciences of,
    104
  guidelines for, 103–104
  importance of, 103
  spiral, 103–106, 105f
  study of, for learning outcomes
    identification, 70
  in task-based learning, clinical
    presentations that provide
    framework for, 275–276
  teaching methods, 99
  transition between courses, 106
  vertically integrated, 24

Curriculum cube, in task-based learning, 121–123, 122f
Customised learning, 208

D

Database, evidence from, 35–36
Decision making strategies, 12
Deliberate practice, simulators and, 198
Delivered curriculum, 92–94, 93f
Delphi technique, 69
Dentistry, tasks mastery grid for vocational training in, 277
Difficulty, increased, in student progression, 271f
Direct observation of procedural skills (DOPS), 241
Directed self-learning, 112, 185
    see also Student-centred learning
Discipline-based learning, 98
Distance learning, 205–206, 206f
Distributed learning, 205–206
    curriculum mapping in, 160
Doctors
    outcome-based education and, 61
    as student assessors, 219
'Dr Fox Effect', 50–51
Dumez, Vincent, 44
Dundee Ready Education Environment Measure (DREEM), 156, 278
Dundee three-circle outcome model, 74–75, 74f

E

Ear, nose and throat, 276
Early clinical experience, 104
Educating Physicians: A Call for Reform of Medical Schools and Residency, 4–5
Education climate, 153–155
'Education for capability', 59
Education for Primary Care, 52
Education programme
    elements of, 3f
    see also Curriculum
The Education Resource Information Centre (ERIC), 35–36
Educational environment, 155–156
    aspects of, 155–156
    assessment of, 156–157
    collaborative or competitive orientation, 155
    community or hospital orientation, 155–156
    and the curriculum, 100–101
    effects of, 156
    importance of, 153–158
    research or teaching orientation, 156
    student or teacher orientation, 155
    supportive or punitive orientation, 155
    use of, 157–158
Educational meetings, evidence from, 35
Educational principles, understanding of, 15–26
Educational researchers, value of curriculum mapping to, 161
Educational strategies, 97–99, 97f
    e-learning, 207–209, 207f
E-learning, 203–209
    blended learning, 206–207
    definition of, 203
    distributed and distance, 205–206, 206f
    educational features of, 204–205
    educational strategies, 207–209, 207f
    a move to, 203
    reasons for introducing, 204
    role of the teacher in, 206
        as an assessor, 205
        as an information provider, 208
        as a curriculum planner, 206
        as a facilitator, 203
        as a role model, 208
Electives, 149
Elective/uniform approach to curriculum, 98
Embase, 35–36
Engaging the audience, 170
Enthusiastic teacher, 27–31
Entrustable Professional Activities (EPAs), 62–65
    curriculum and, 64–65
    definition of, 62–63
    granularity and, 63, 63f
    learner outcomes and competencies, 63–64, 63f
    specification of level of supervision and, 64
Entrustable Professional Activities (EPAS), for undergraduate medical education, 268
Environment, educational, 155–156
    aspects of, 155–156
    assessment of, 156–157
    collaborative or competitive orientation, 155
    community or hospital orientation, 155–156
    and the curriculum, 100–101
    effects of, 156
    importance of, 153–158
    research or teaching orientation, 156
    student or teacher orientation, 155
    supportive or punitive orientation, 155
    use of, 157–158
Errors in practice, studies of, 70
Essay questions, 233

Essential Skills in Medical Education, 52
Ethics, 12
Evidence
    definition of, 35
    evaluating for, 36–37
    searching for, 35–36
'Evidence-based curriculum', 34
Evidence-based medicine (EBM), 34
Evidence-informed teaching, 34–35
Examiners
    in clinical and performance-based assessment, 242–243
    in portfolio assessment, 249–250
Exchange-based learning, 133
Exit outcomes, 57
Experience, early clinical, 104
Experience-based learning. see Work-based learning.
Extended matching questions (EMQs), 234–235
Eyes, 276

F

Facilitators, teachers as, 9–10
    in e-learning, 203
FAIR acronym, 15, 16f
Feasibility of student assessment tools, 225
Feedback, 16–18
    in clinical and performance-based assessment, 243–244
    definition of, 17
    multi-source, 241–242
    obtaining, from colleagues, 51
    providing
        basic principles, 15
        technical skills for, 11
    provision of, 18
    student assessment as, 221
Fever and infection, 275
Fidelity of simulators, 200
Flipped classroom, 18, 171–174
    advantages and disadvantages of, 172–173
    comparison of the traditional lecture and, 172f
    definition of, 171–172
    implementation in practice, 173–174
    medical education, application in, 172
Focus group technique, 69
Frameworks, of learning outcomes, 73
    criteria for, 73
Fried, R.L., 27
The Future of Medical Education in Canada (FMEC): A Collective Vision for MD Education, 4–5
The Future of Medical Education in Scotland, 4

G

Garland, Peter, 104
General Medical Council, 4, 77–79
  expectations for learning
    outcomes, 67
General mental ability test, 256
Global Independent Commission on
  Education of Health Professionals,
  154–155
Global Minimum Essential
  Requirements (GMER), 77
Globalisation, 204
Goldacre, 34
Good, Thomas, 3–4
Good teacher, 1
  different faces of, 9–13
  as professional, 12–13
  range of abilities of, 9–11, 10f
  requirements of, 9
  technical competencies of, 10f, 11
  work approach of, 11–12
Graduates
  assessment of, for curriculum
    evaluation, 262
  interviews with, for learning
    outcomes identification, 70
  selection for entry to medicine,
    254
Granularity, Entrustable Professional
  Activities and, 63, 63f
Guides
  keeping up to date from, 52
  see also Study guides

H

Handouts at lecture, 171
Harmonisation, integration
  continuum, 128
Harvey cardiac simulator, 198f, 200,
  238
Health care professionals,
  collaboration with, 44
Hidden curriculum, 92–94
Horizontal integration, 126
Hospital orientation, in education
  environment, 155–156
Hospital-based learning, 98

I

Independent learning, 183–187
  benefits for student, 184
  in curriculum, 184–185
    directed self-learning and role of
      teacher, 185
    study guides for, 185, 186f
    time allocated for, and
      scheduling in, 184–185
  importance of, 183–184
  learning resources for, 186–187

Individualisation, of students, 15,
  20–23, 21f
Individualised learning, simulators
  and, 198
'Inert knowledge', 19
'Information explosion', 145
Information overload, 24, 145–151
  advantages of core curriculum
    with SSCs, 146–147, 147f
  core curriculum with options or
    student-selected components,
    146
  problem of, 145, 145f
  responding to problem, 146
  threshold concepts, 148–149
Information providers, teachers as,
  9–10
  in e-learning, 208
Information-orientated learning, 98
Information-oriented approach,
  summary of various points in
  continuum between problem-
  based approach and, 273–274
Institutions, assessment of, 260
Integrated approach, use of, 125–130
Integrated curriculum, move to,
  125–126, 125f
Integrated learning, curriculum
  mapping in, 160
Integrated/discipline-based learning,
  98
Integration
  advantages of, 126–127
  of assessment and teaching,
    curriculum mapping in, 160
  continuum, 127–130, 128f
  focus for, 127
Intentional learning, 208
Inter-disciplinary, integration
  continuum, 129
International Competency-Based
  Medical Education (ICBME), 58
International dimensions, 204
International Institute for Medical
  Education, learning outcomes,
  67
Interprofessional education (IPE),
  131–134
  continuum of, 132
  curriculum mapping in, 160
  implementation in practice,
    132–134
  implementation strategy in, 133
  move to, 131
  tackling a negative mindset,
    133–134
  vision for, 132
Interprofessional learning, principles
  of, 131–132
Interviews, selection for entry to
  medicine, 256
Intuition, 38–39
Isolation, integration continuum, 127
'Ivory Tower', 90–91

J

Journal club, 177
Journals, keeping up to date from, 52

K

Keeping up to date, 49–54
Key topics, outcome-based education
  and, 59
Kirkpatrick's four levels of curriculum
  evaluation, 263–264, 264f
Knowledge, mastery of, 223

L

Large group. see Lectures.
Learned curriculum, 92–94, 93f
Learning, in clinical problems and
  presentations, 117–123
Learning environment, 153
Learning from practice. see
  Work-based learning.
Learning opportunity, independent
  learning and, 185
Learning outcomes
  approaches for, 69–71
  in clinical and performance-based
    assessment, 242
  communicating, 73–79
  for competent practitioner,
    269–270
  describing, 73–79
  different phases of education and,
    68f
  expected, from the curriculum, 96
  first two sections of, 277
  frameworks for, 73
    criteria for, 73
  involvement of stakeholders in,
    68–69
  in small group work, 179
  specification of, 67–71
  and student assessment, 223
  through small group teaching,
    175–176
  see also Outcome-based education
    (OBE)
Learning resources
  independent, 20
  in independent learning, 186–187
  in outcome-based education, 60
  technical competencies of
    teachers in using, 11
Lecture theatre, 181–182
Lectures, 167–174
  active learning in, 19
  delivering good, 168–171
    close of the lecture, 170–171
    content and structure, 169
    engaging the audience, 170
    getting facts in advance, 169

handouts, 171
introduction, 169
visual aids, 170
flipped classroom, 171–174
presence and behaviour at, 171
problems with, 167–168, 168f
technical skills for, 11
traditional, comparison of flipped
classroom and, 172f
use of, 167
when to use, 168
Life cycle, integrated learning of, 127
Life threatening/accident and
emergency, 276
Literature, evidence from, 35
Longitudinal integrated clerkships
(LICs), 135–143
features of, 138
implementation of, 138
traditional clinical clerkships,
problem with, 137–138
Lumps, bumps and swelling, 275

M

Manager, teachers as, 9–10
Manikins
in clinical and performance-based
assessment, 238
in simulation, 196
Massive open online courses
(MOOCs), 206
Mastery of knowledge, 223
McAuliffe, Christa, 6
McLean, Michelle, 35
Medical advances, and outcome-
based education, 59
Medical education
accountability and transparency
in, outcome-based education
and, 59–60
changes in, 5t
courses on, keeping up to date
from, 52
different phases of, collaboration
between, 42–44
important trend in, 57
Medical Education, 52
Medical school
collaboration between teachers
within, 42
vision/mission of, 95–96
Medical Science Education, 52
Medical Teacher, 35, 52
Medicine
changes in, curriculum mapping
in, 160
rapid advances in, outcome-based
education and, 59
Medline, 35–36
Meetings, keeping up to date from,
52
Miller, George, 27

Miller's pyramid, 237, 238f
Mini clinical evaluation exercise
(Mini-CEX), 240–241
Mixed economy, 70–71
Models
in clinical and performance-based
assessment, 238
in simulation, 197–199
Modified essay questions (MEQs), 235
Multi-disciplinary, integration
continuum, 129
Multiple choice questions (MCQs),
234
Multiple mini-interview (MMI), 256
Multi-source feedback (MSF),
241–242

N

Nesting, integration continuum, 128
New York Commission on Medical
Education, 42
Newsletters, keeping up to date
from, 52
Nominal group technique, 69
Non-threatening environment,
simulators and, 199
Norm-referenced approach to
student assessment, 221
Nutrition/weight, 275

O

Objective structured clinical
examination (OSCE), 16, 51, 100,
239–240, 247–248
stations, examples of, 279
Objective structured long
examination record (OSLER), 239
Objective Structured Teaching
Exercise (OSTE), 51
Observation-based learning, 133
Online information, keeping up to
date from, 52
On-the-job learning (OJL). *see*
Work-based learning.
Opportunistic learning, 99
Ostriches, outcome-based education
implementation, 81
Outcome-based approach,
implementation of
ostriches, peacocks and beavers,
81
in practice, 81–85
Outcome-based education (OBE), 57,
81
advantages of, 59–61
concept of, 57
curriculum, student progression in,
82
curriculum mapping in, 160
definition of, 57–59, 58f

features of, 62b
implementation of, 67
guidelines of, 82–83
inventory, 83–85, 84f
programme, 81–82
myths and concerns about,
61–62
Outcome/competency-based
approach, 59–61
move to, 57–65

P

P2P learning, 211
benefits of, 212–213
definition of, 211
examples of, 212
implementation in practice,
213–214
recognition of, 211
Pain, 275–276
Paralysis and impaired mobility, 275
Passionate teacher, 27–31, 29f
The Passionate Teacher, 27
Patient(s)
in clinical and performance-based
assessment, 237–239
'real', 238
role in clinical teaching, 191–192
simulated, 196–197, 238
standardised, 196
virtual, 199–200
Peacocks, outcome-based education
implementation, 81
Peer evaluation, 223
Peer learning, 211–216
benefits of, 212–213
examples of, 212
implementation in practice,
213–216
Peer-assisted learning, 99
Performance at school, 255
Personal development, 50
Personal experience, evidence from,
35
Personality inventories, 257
'PHOG' approach, 33–34, 33f
Planned curriculum, 92–94, 93f, 99,
259
Planners, teachers as, 9–10
in e-learning, 206
Planning
clinical teaching, 192–193
curriculum
in problem-based learning, 119
questions to ask when, 95–101
trends in, 135
Portfolio assessment, 247–251
advantages of, 248
definition of, 247
implementation of, 249–251
Portfolio learning, active learning
from, 19–20

Postgraduate Hospital Education Environment Measure (PHEEM), 157
Postgraduate training
and clinical teaching, 190
environment, 154
selection for entry to, 253–258
PowerPoint, 170
A Practical Guide for Medical Teachers, 52
Practitioner, learning outcomes for, 269–270
Prerequisites, 103
Presentations, technical skills for, 11
Priority setting, decision making and audit, 276
Problem-assisted learning, 273–274
Problem-based approach, continuum between information-oriented approach and, summary of various points in, 273–274
Problem-based learning (PBL), 98, 118–119, 273–274
context for, 119
continuum of, 119
curriculum mapping in, 160
in small groups, 178
Problem-based mixed approach, 273–274
Problem-centred discovery learning, 273–274
Problem-centred learning, 273–274
Problem-focused learning, 273–274
Problem-initiated learning, 273–274
Problem-orientated learning, 273–274
Problem-solving learning, 273–274
Professional development, 272f
Professional education associations, keeping up to date from, 52–53
Professionalism, 50
concept of, to teaching, 10
Proficiency, increased, in student progression, 271f
PsycINFO, 35–36
Published review/guide/editorial, evidence from, 35
Punitive orientation, in education environment, 155

Q

QUESTS criteria, 36–37

R

Received curriculum, 259
References, selection for entry to medicine, 255–256
Reflection, in active learning, 19
Relevance, of learning, 15, 23–26
Reliability of student assessment tools, 224–225, 224f, 248

Repetitive practice, simulators and, 198
Reports, keeping up to date from, 52
Reproductive problems, 276
Research orientation, in education environment, 156
Researchers, educational, value of curriculum mapping to, 161
'Results-orientated thinking', 57
see also Outcome-based education (OBE)
Role models, teachers as, 9–10
in e-learning, 208
Role-playing, 177
Royal College of Physicians and Surgeons, 67
Rural setting, 136–137

S

Scholar, teachers as, 9–10
Scholarship, in teaching, 53–54
Scholarship Reconsidered, 12–13
School, performance at, 255
School leavers, selection for entry to medicine, 254
Schools, medical
assessment of, 259
mission of, 260
The 'Scottish Doctor' framework, 74–75, 74f
Script concordance test (SCT), 235
Selection for entry to medicine, 253–258
aims of, 254
choice of, 255–258
criteria for, 254–255
importance of, 253
Self-assessment, 19, 205
Self-directed learning, 112, 185
see also Student-centred learning
Seminar, 177
Senior house officers, training guide for, 272
Sequencing of courses, 103
Service-based learning. see Work-based learning.
Settings
clinical. see Clinical setting
teaching in a variety of, 11
urban and rural, 136–137
Sharing, integration continuum, 128
Short answer questions (SAQs), 234
Short essay questions (SEQs), 233–234
Simulated patients, 196–197
in clinical and performance-based assessment, 238
recruiting and training, 197
Simulation, 195–202
active learning from, 19–20
choice of, 200
of clinical experience, 195–202

clinical skills centres, 200–202
computer-based, 239
reasons for, 195–196
simulated patients. see Simulated patients
simulating 'real' patients, 196
simulators (manikins and models), 197–199, 198f
virtual patients, 199–200
advantages of using, 199–200
uses of, 199
Simulation-based learning, 133
Simulators, 196
availability, 200
in clinical and performance-based assessment, 238
fidelity of, 200
Situated learning. see Work-based learning.
Situational judgement tests (SJTs), 235, 256
Skin problems, 275
Small group, learning in, 175–182
Small group teaching
active learning, in, 19
advantages of, 176
definition of, 175
implementing, 178–180
before activity, 178–179, 179f
during activity, 179–180
after the activity, 180
problems with, 176–177
role of, 175–176
role of teacher in, 178
technical skills for, 11
techniques used in, 177–178
Snowballing, 177
'Spaced learning', 104–105
Spady, W.G., 57
Specialty training, selection for admission to, 257–258
SPICES model, 97–98, 97f
Spiral curriculum, 103–106, 105f
Stakeholders
collaboration with, 44
involvement in learning outcomes, 68–69
Standard setting
student assessment, 226
written examinations, 233
Standardised patient, 196
Stress, 30–31
Structured learning, 208
Student assessment
clinical and performance-based, 237–245
approaches to, 239–242
considerations in, 221
the examiner in, 220f, 242–243
importance of, 219–220, 237
the patient in, 237–239
portfolio, 242
competence, 237
competency-based, 224

computer-based. *see* Written and computer-based assessment
criterion-referenced approach to, 221
deciding what should be assessed, 221
formative, 221
location of, 228–229
norm-referenced approach to, 221
outcome-based education and, 60
portfolio, 247–251
  advantages of, 248
  definition of, 247
  implementation of, 249–251
problems with, 219
programmatic, 226–227
progress test, 227–228
reasons for, 223
selection for entry to medicine, 253–258
stakeholders in, 219
standard setting, 226
summative, 221
technical skills for, 11
timing of, 227
tools/instruments for, 224–226, 224*f*
written and computer-based, 231–236, 232*f*
  elements in, 231–233
  role of, 231
  technology, 235–236
  types of, 233–235
Student-centred approach, student engagement and, 109–114
Student-centred learning, 98
adaptive learning, 112–113
curriculum mapping in, 160
definition of, 111–114
move from teacher-centred to, 109, 110*f*, 111*t*
power relationship from teacher to student, shift of, 113–114
reasons for, 109–110
responsibility for, 111–112, 112*b*
role of the teacher, 109
use of study guides in, 112
Student(s), 3–4, 3*f*
assessment of. *see* Student assessment
being FAIR to, 15–16
benefits of independent learning, 184
engagement, and student- centred approach, 109–114
four dimensions of progression, 271
learning, 55
  clinical problem in, importance of, 117
mobility, curriculum mapping and, 160
motivating, use of assessment in, 222

orientation, in education environment, 155
outcome-based education and, 60
profile, in clinical and performance-based assessment, 243, 243*f*
progression, 192
  in OBE curriculum, 82
references, 255–256
responsibility for learning, 111–112, 112*b*
role in clinical teaching, 190
value of curriculum mapping to, 161
Student-selected components, 146, 149
advantages of core curriculum with, 146–147, 147*f*
assessment of, 150
choice of topics, 149–150
integration of, with the core, 150–151
Study guides
elements of, 112
in independent learning, 185, 186*f*
use in student-centred learning, 112
Support staff, value of curriculum mapping to, 161
Supportive orientation, in education environment, 155
Surgery theatre educational environment measure (STEEM), 157
Systematic/ apprenticeship approach to learning, 99
Systematic reviews
evidence from, 35
keeping up to date from, 52

T

Task analysis, 70
Task-based learning (TkBL), 119–123, 120*f*, 273–274
clinical presentation of, 121
in clinical setting, 120
curriculum cube, 121–123, 122*f*
curriculum planning, 98
definition of, 119–120, 120*f*
framework for curriculum in, 275–276
implementation of, 120–121
Tasks mastery grid, for vocational training in dentistry, 277
Teacher-centred learning
curriculum planning, 98
move to student-centred, 109, 110*f*, 111*t*
Teacher(s), 3–4, 3*f*
burn out of, 30–31
collaboration between

for local, national, international programme, 44–45
within medical school, 42
curriculum, student and, 3–4, 3*f*
enthusiastic, 27–31
good, 1
  different faces of, 9–13
  as professional, 12–13
  range of abilities of, 9–11, 10*f*
  requirements of, 9
  technical competencies of, 10*f*, 11
  work approach of, 11–12
importance of, 3–7
motivation of, 6–7
necessary attributes, 4–6, 5*t*
orientation, in education environment, 155
outcome-based education and, 60–61
passionate, 27–31, 29*f*
roles of
  in clinical teaching, 190, 191*t*
  in e-learning, 206
  in problem-based learning, 118–119
  in small group work, 178
  in student-centred learning, 109
stress of, 30–31
toolkit, 99
value of curriculum mapping to, 160–161
Teaching, 10
evidence-informed, 34–35
judgement, intuition and, 38–39
motivation for, 6–7
orientation, in education environment, 156
passion in, 28
as professional activity, 49–50, 49*f*
scholarship of, 12–13, 53–54
styles of, 165
Teaching and Learning in Medicine, 52
Team, collaborating and working as, 41–47
Team-based learning (TBL), 180–182
definition of, 180
implementation of, 181–182
Teamwork, 272*f*
Technical competencies, of good teacher, 10*f*, 11
Technology, written and computer-based assessment, 235–236
Temporal coordination, integration continuum, 128
Ten questions framework, for curriculum evaluation, 261–263
Textbooks, keeping up to date from, 52
'The Scottish Doctor' report, 67–68
Theoretical learning, 273–274
Therapy, 272*f*

360 degrees evaluation, 241–242
Three-circle outcome model, 74–75, 74f
  learning outcomes for a competent practitioner based on, 269–270
Threshold concepts, 96, 148–149
  importance of, 149
  key characteristics of, 148–149
  responding to information overload and building options into a core curriculum with, 145–151
Tomorrow's Doctors, 67
Tosteson, Dan, 4
Traditional clinical clerkships, problem with, 137–138
Training, postgraduate
  and clinical teaching, 190
  environment, 154
  selection for entry to, 253–258
Training programme, vision/mission of, 95–96
Trans-disciplinary, integration continuum, 129–130

Transition between courses, 106
Transparency, outcome-based education and, 59–60
Tutorial, 177

U

Undergraduate medical education, Entrustable Professional Activities (EPAS) for, 268
Uniform approach, to curriculum, 98
Urban setting, 136–137
Utility, increased, in student progression, 271f

V

Validity of student assessment tools, 225, 225f, 248
Van der Vleuten, Cees, 33
Vertical integration, 126
Virtual patients
  active learning from, 20

advantages of, 199–200
definition of, 199–200
Visual aids in lecture, 170
Vocational training, tasks mastery grid for, in dentistry, 277

W

Whitehead, A.N., 27
Work-based learning, 138–143
  advantages of, 139
  definition of, 138–139
  implementation of, 140–141, 140f
  principles of, 139
  problems and pitfalls of, 141–143, 141f
Worley, Paul, 35
Written and computer-based assessment, 231–236, 232f
  elements in, 231–233
  role of, 231
  technology, 235–236
  types of, 233–235